Sociology in Practice for Health Care Professionals

Ron Iphofen
and
Fiona Poland

Consultant editor: Jo Campling

MACMILLAN

First published 1998 by
MACMILLAN PRESS LTD
Houndmills, Basingstoke, Hampshire RG21 6XS
and London
Companies and representatives
throughout the world

ISBN 0–333–64576–6 paperback

A catalogue record for this book is available
from the British Library.

This book is printed on paper suitable for recycling and
made from fully managed and sustained forest sources.

10 9 8 7 6 5 4 3 2 1
07 06 05 04 03 02 01 00 99 98

Editing and origination by
Aardvark Editorial, Mendham, Suffolk

Printed in Malaysia

Contents

Preface: How To Use This Book

One of our reasons for writing this book was to offer an alternative to the more academic introductions to the discipline of sociology. We are assuming that you, our readers, are health care professionals or students who need to use sociology to improve the quality of the care that you give. We hope you are reading the book to broaden your knowledge of your clients and of yourselves. We offer you routes to reflect on action from a sociological viewpoint.

The emphasis of this book is on showing how, starting from your own personal situation, you can begin to locate and use resources which support health and caring. We are also concerned to analyse the constraints on health and care work across a range of social settings. In focusing on the practical experience of health care professionals we look at the exercise of power and oppression within informal and formal care settings. We look at the inequalities which underlie the everyday lives of those working as partners in different kinds of health care encounters: the professional, the carer and the cared-for. We want to highlight the importance of everyday ways of coming to know about health settings and issues.

Small sections of the text are highlighted in bold – **like this**. By doing this we hope to draw your attention to issues and concepts which we believe are particularly important. Next to each section of bold text there will be an explanation or comment which clarifies its importance. The ideas we present are cumulative so that we do not recommend reading chapters out of context. We are trying to build your expertise with the means and methods of sociological analysis which are of value in health care practice. For example, fully understanding what we say about health policy in Chapter 14 requires understanding the issues of power and inequality which we deal with in Chapters 2 and 7.

There is no separate glossary of terms. We define each new concept as simply as possible when we introduce it. If you want to know more about each idea, use a dictionary or encyclopaedia of sociology. Treat this as a **workbook**, with ideas, observations and exercises of relevance to practice. It is not intended as a comprehensive sociology textbook. There are many good basic sociology texts which you could use to supplement the work you do in response to our suggestions. Look at the **further reading** sections at the end of each chapter if you wish to follow up on any ideas.

We believe that reading and learning are best done **actively**. You should always have in mind your own sense of **relevance** – why *you* are reading this book, why *you* are studying this subject, what knowledge or information *you* hope to gain, how *you* can use this knowledge in your practice, what problems *you* hope to solve.

Exercise

Before starting this book try writing a brief description of how you see your future professional care work. Write about the tasks you anticipate doing, where you will be working, the sort of behaviour you engage in or expect to engage in, and how you expect to feel. Write honestly, since this material is the basic resource with which you relate to this book.

There are **Exercises** and **Key Questions** in boxes, just like the one above, which we ask you to do to encourage you to develop these ideas further. They are designed to keep you intellectually active as you read, to encourage reflection and to build your skills in sociological analysis. **Please do not skip over these boxes**. Put the book down and **write the answers** to the questions. Such writing will form the basis of what you learn and will inform your future practice.

Similarly, relate other reading and writing to the ideas which we raise. Take note of popular ideas about health and illness that you come across on television or in the newspapers. Keep a cuttings file of interesting articles, or letters to the newspaper. Sociology can then be used to show how your clients' and your own imagery about health care is generated, and to analyse how appropriate that imagery is and how it might change.

The best way to learn from sociology is to treat it as an intellectual adventure, a voyage involving discovery, thought, dialogue and imagination. Enjoy the trip.

Acknowledgements

We would like to thank all our students and health care professional colleagues, past and present, who have tried out the exercises contained here. We have made amendments based on their comments. The guidance and patience shown by Jo Campling and Catherine Gray at Macmillan are sincerely appreciated. We would particularly like to acknowledge the research assistance of Carol Iphofen; in addition, her reading and commentary on drafts immensely improved the lucidity of what we wanted to say.

Chapter 1 The Nature of Sociology: Explanations and Applications

Health and illness affect not just people's bodies, but also how they organise their whole lives: working, relaxing, caring and feeling in control. Health care professionals have to **care for the whole person**, which means avoiding treating people as a set of body parts or symptoms. Professionals need methods for understanding their clients, their colleagues and themselves. Sociology is about **understanding the individual's place in the world**: where they are, what they do and what their views are. It is about how they come to be in that place and think the things that they think.

Understanding is not the same as being sympathetic nor is it concerned with making moral judgements about people's situations; it has everything to do with explanation. Likes or dislikes, prejudices or stereotypes, cannot be allowed to determine client care. For care to be effective, carers must keep in mind the particular features which affect each client's social situation.

You do not have to be a brilliant sociologist to make use of sociology as a health care professional. It is one of several disciplines which can offer useful insights into your professional practice and it is used in a similar way in a wide range of other professions. Sociology helps to understand the influences on you and on your clients, influences which condition behaviour, beliefs and attitudes.

Sociology is a **scientific** discipline. Being scientific means that sociologists can rigorously and thoroughly review each other's work and make judgements about whether or not a piece of research makes a genuine contribution to knowledge. However, sociology is also a **discursive** discipline which draws on common sense because that is our basic data: how people see and experience the world. Common sense is not always sensible and rational, but it is what people use to guide their lives.

One of the qualities that sociology needs is detachment. This means moving beyond the personal assumptions and concerns of doing and surviving a job. You will find that sociological insights can help with that very survival by examining the processes people use to manage their everyday lives and by offering a variety of means for dealing with difficult situations.

In the same way sociology can help you as a professional to understand your own place in the world. The health care professions are going through an exciting but difficult time of change in which there is much disagreement about their roles. Some means of detachment will enable you to ask useful questions about what you experience.

Common difficulties with the discipline

1. Sociology is not easy. It can be abstract and diverse. It is conceptually difficult since writers use different terms and it is not easy to question the routines and assumptions that we take for granted. You need patience, a recognition that all disciplines have their own special language and a willingness to make use of a good sociological dictionary.

2. Sociology does not offer clear solutions to society's problems. It exists to explain society. Explanation can help us to make constructive reform and sensible social policies. However, social policies are designed and implemented by politicians, by civil servants and by what professionals do in practice.

3. When studying crime and social deviance sociologists are often accused of siding with the offender and ignoring the victim. In fact, both are studied in great detail, but the explanation for why a crime has happened is not always found in the behaviour of the victim. Much time has to be spent studying offenders. Moreover, to explain why a crime happened is not to condone or excuse it. Sociologists avoid taking sides when conducting their analysis.

4. Another misconception is that sociologists often suggest that different health opportunities, poverty, unemployment and so

on are a consequence of conspiracy. On the whole, sociologists do not think that inequality is a consequence of a deliberate plan to keep people ignorant and in their place. Rather, they believe that social structures emerge as a result of the independent decisions and behaviour of individuals across society. Some people are more powerful than others, but they do not all collude with one another. Nonetheless, their separate actions produce inequalities. What matters is finding out why people take such decisions in the first place, how inequalities emerge and what consequences they have for behaviour.

Healthy and unhealthy behaviour

We illustrate these points with a few examples. The following incidents are true. Take time to think about them and write notes to explain why they took place. Our explanations follow.

Exercise

1. An old woman has fallen in a ditch. People stand by and watch her die, although they could help her out. After she dies they share out her belongings between them.

2. A mother assists in holding down her nine-year-old daughter while friends and neighbours cut out the daughter's clitoris and labia.

3. A mother sits on a couch gently massaging her two-year-old daughter's clitoris while she sits on her knee.

4. People self-administer poisons which they know will harm them.

---

1. This story is taken from observations of a tribe called the Ik in North East Uganda in the 1960s. The region was extremely impoverished. The death of an old person benefited the younger, healthier members of the tribe. They did not deliberately kill the old woman, but neither did they feel any moral responsibility to help her. It was for the greatest good of the greatest number that they did not help her to live.

2. This sounds to many of us like child abuse, but female circumcision happens to eighty million women a year in Africa alone. It has a long history. Women who do it and who have had it done are often proud of it as morally right and proper. It signifies their chastity and propriety. Although women maintain the practice, one explanation is that it keeps them in their place as the property of men. If they are unable to have any sexual pleasure, it is argued that they are unlikely to be unfaithful. Only in recent years has the practice been criticised.

3. This incident was observed in a British middle-class family nearly thirty years ago. When questioned by the observer the mother replied that it helped the child to relax and to sleep. Today this practice might not have been observed because of public awareness of child sexual abuse. At the time the mother clearly thought there was no harm in it, otherwise she would not have done it publicly. It is also clear that the mother did not have any abusive intent; it was done therapeutically. This may have been done to the mother herself in infancy as a practice in her own family. Did it do the child any harm at the time? Does the child now suffer, in maturity, as a result of heightened public concern with child abuse?

4. Apart from attempts to self-harm or to commit suicide people in many cultures do this in work or leisure. Mexican Indians take mescaline in peyote, a drug which induces psychosis or schizophrenia and which does not break down in the body. In the West people regularly take painkillers which damage the kidneys. Some men in the UK drink fifteen pints of beer a night. People all over the world smoke tobacco, overeat, engage in dangerous exercise, work in hazardous occupations and so on.

Such examples show that people routinely do apparently unhealthy things – practices which do not enhance their health. If we rely on common sense alone, we cannot explain these things; the reasons for people behaving in such ways are much more complex. People do these things for social, cultural, economic, political, and psychological reasons. Humans are not dominated by their biology or their physiology. Physiology dictates that humans need to eat, sleep, seek warmth, seek shelter and indulge in sex, and that they can see, hear, touch, taste and think. They do these things all over the world – but not in the same ways. How and why they differ is a social phenomenon. These things can only be explained by studying them on a variety of levels: on the levels of culture, economics, politics, biology, physiology and so on. Sociology offers **one level of explanation** among many. To study any piece of human behaviour fully requires that we put all the different levels of explanation together. This is what is meant by **holism**: understanding human actions, thoughts and beliefs in terms of *all* the influences on us. At times those who believe in the importance of a particular level of explanation have advocated a **reductionist** approach, suggesting, for example, that we can 'reduce' the understanding of all human action to some basic physiological or psychological drive. Sociology tends toward more holistic explanations, striving towards the fullest possible account of human behaviour.

In recent years medical explanations have become more holistic, drawing more often on the social and behavioural sciences. Health care professionals recognise that people have health problems as a result of their activities, but they cannot explain why the incidents occurred without some sociologically based explanation. Even when we can explain such events, and provide care for the individuals who suffer, this does not mean that we can solve the underlying problem. Knowing why and how things happen does not in itself solve the problem. People have to confront problems and then engage in social and political solutions.

To be a modern health care professional you must ask yourself uncomfortable questions if you are to cultivate a critical awareness of social influences on health behaviour and on the origins and consequences of illness.

Ordinary life

The examples given above are chosen to emphasise a point. Most sociological concerns are more mundane than these, much closer to our shared experiences. We need to **see even the mundane as out of the ordinary** in order to detach ourselves from simply living it. We should be able to examine and question even behaviour which we consider to be 'normal' and 'healthy'.

Consider some things we tend to take for granted, such as working, sleeping and eating. Many people in the West consider breakfast to be important before leaving the house for work. They often have a cold light lunch and have a main meal in the evening after returning home from work. They try to sleep eight hours a night throughout the year.

Yet such a routine is relatively recent. Until the early nineteenth century the main hot meal was taken at midday. Most people worked at home and, in the winter, slept for longer. The organisation of work and life was more in accord with natural biological rhythms. Industrialisation and the growth of the factory system interfered with this. Far more people left their homes for work, to spend long hours at their job and to eat and sleep as factory hours permitted. While the wealthier classes were able to retain the traditional customs, the working classes were more at the mercy of changes in the structure of work. This accounts for variations in eating and working patterns between the classes even today.

An interesting cultural contrast is provided by sleeping after lunch. People take a siesta in Spain and parts of Central and South America. Some business executives now advocate a ten minute 'power-nap' during the working day.

Exercise

Ask questions about behaviour which seems ordinary to you.

Make a note of some of your own routines. How long have you being doing them? Why did you start to do things that way in the first place? If they change, why do they do so?

Social problems

Between these examples of ordinary behaviour and the more unusual incidents lie issues connected with contemporary social problems. Many problems seem to occur repetitively, giving cause for concern and having implications for health behaviour and attitudes. These include fashion or diet victims, sexual harassment, domestic violence, football hooliganism, homelessness and crime.

It is difficult to set the boundaries between the normal, the problematic and the unusual. What is normal or routine for us may be unusual to someone else, but any of the behaviour described above could have implications for human health. We should question what is healthy about routine behaviour such as sleeping, eating and working. What is healthy about what we eat, how we eat, where and when we sleep, or how and why we work? Is normal behaviour healthy? Why and how do we take exercise? Why do we go on holiday, play tennis or darts and so on? Raising issues like those above does call our complacency into question.

This is what sociology does. Our aim is to encourage and develop an ability to engage in informed, rigorous and objective analysis of social issues. You may not alter your own prejudices, attitudes or emotional reactions, but you will at least better understand how you come to hold certain views and also how your clients and colleagues come to be the people that they are.

Theories and perspectives

We cannot perform such an analysis without some guidelines. It is here that the theories put forward by sociologists are useful. Theories offer us a framework within which to interpret our observations and experiences. By thinking in terms of the patterns or structures of the social world, theories can help us make sense of the sorts of example we gave earlier. While sociology is neither social policy nor social engineering, it is the case that the solutions to social problems require action. Action is misguided if it is not properly informed. Informed action depends upon adequate explanation.

Exercise

The question 'What is going on here?' is essentially theoretical and can be applied to any event or social setting. Ask it of a learning situation – in a classroom or a library; of a professional/client encounter; of the routine interactions which take place within your household. One way to do this is to imagine you are a visitor from another planet. You first try to describe what you see and then attempt to explain it. So you need to answer some of the following questions:

● What behaviour is being engaged in?

cont'd

- Who is in the group (including physically obvious variations such as gender, age, size and colour)?
- How do they relate to each other?
- What things appear to influence them?
- What are the consequences of this behaviour?
- What action needs to be taken (if any)?

Think in terms of...

first, **describing** the situation or event;

then, **explaining** why the things you describe are happening;

next, **predicting** what might happen in such settings in the future;

and, finally, discussing what sorts of policy or direct **action** might be used.

You can probably do this already if you are a keen observer of people. Our aim is to improve your skills at such tasks, and to encourage you to look more deeply into human relationships and the structures within which they occur so that, ultimately, you will become a more effective health care professional.

Theories have to be useful for explaining the world and people's places in it. To be more than just common sense they have to be testable and to be tested. In this sense theories are distinguished from ideologies. An **ideology** is a co-ordinated set of beliefs about the nature of the world, but beliefs rely on faith and, as such, are often hard to change even in the light of evidence which contradicts them. People tend to hold on to their ideologies with conviction. This should not happen with theories which should be subject to change in the light of new knowledge or new evidence. For example, throughout history there have been changes in the theoretical views of the human body and how it functions, the organic world and the origins of the universe.

Nonetheless, there are links between theories and ideologies. Both are abstract and therefore metaphorical. They **re-present** what is going on the world, but they are not the world – just as 'a map is not the territory'. Ideologies often extract ideas from theories in order to justify certain beliefs. For example, the Nazis drew ideas from genetics to advocate the supremacy of one race

8

over all the others. For now we will concentrate on theories, but we will make reference to ideologies as we proceed and return to look at ideologies and their consequences in more detail in Chapter 11.

Main perspectives in sociology

There are various theoretical perspectives which are central to sociology. Each theory has been developed within the context of the social and cultural concerns of the time, yet each still has relevance to our understanding of the modern world.

One of the earliest social theories was **functionalism**. The simplest of the many varieties of functionalist theory was the **organic analogy**, which emerged in the late nineteenth century in the work of Herbert Spencer. Its origins were linked to ideas about human evolution and to the success of Charles Darwin's views. This theory argued that society has (like organisms) certain functions to be performed. Reproduction, the care and education of the young and the control of all members of the group are unavoidable tasks which have to be accomplished by any society if it is to survive. These functions are performed by **social institutions** such as the family, education and the law. It was assumed that, when such functions were performed properly, society would be 'healthy'; if not, various kinds of social pathology would occur.

Through applying this analogy theories about social evolution were constructed. Societies were assumed to be at different levels of development. The more developed societies were seen as superior to others – just as there are higher forms of animal life. Similarly, the idea of natural selection and the survival of the fittest makes it acceptable to allow human organisations to find their own level and this was used to justify *laissez-faire*/free market philosophies.

In the 1940s and 50s sociologists became interested in extending functionalism into **systems theory**. From this perspective all societies and social processes are viewed as if they were systems which were deliberately designed to achieve specific purposes. Talcott Parsons (1951), for example, argued that systems have *inputs* and *outputs* and mechanisms by which the inputs are dealt with. Health care systems have been viewed like this in terms of inputs (admissions) and outputs (discharges). Social institutions are represented as if they resembled a large 'machine'.

Other theories present society as being not integrated like a machine but in conflict. The most significant of such **conflict theorists** was Karl Marx. Marx assumed that people formed groups according to how they related to **limited and unfairly distributed resources**. Some people were seen as owners and controllers of important resources; others had no resources, so had to do as they were told in order to survive. Fundamentally, these groups were in conflict since their interests did not coincide. Marx argued that the underdogs – who were in the majority – would only take this for so long. This conflict of interest would have to be resolved, more than likely in some form of revolution. The basic reason for this conflict was seen to be **capitalism** – an economic system driven by the profit motive. This theory argued that people act in their own interests. The interests of different groups in society – including their health interests – do not always coincide. Health, being a scarce resource, is something that those who own and control tend to have most of, so the poorer members of society are less likely to be healthy.

Both functionalism and Marxist conflict theory are **structuralist** perspectives in emphasising how large, social structures tend to constrain the actions of individuals. From a functionalist viewpoint there is an inevitability about being members of a social institution such as a family even though people choose individually to marry and have children. Similarly, from a conflict perspective, we have to exist in society either as a member of the owner classes or as a member of the working classes and will thus find ourselves socially constrained in either case. We are constrained not only when we do not have resources, but also when we have the responsibilities of owning them.

Interactionist perspectives emerged in the early twentieth century and focused on understanding small groups and individual interactions in terms of how people speak and the signs and symbols they construct. One of the earliest advocates of this perspective, G.H. Mead, argued that language and gestures, as forms of symbolic communication, have a mediating role *between* people. People always try to make sense of their situation. They strive to understand the meanings contained in language, signs and symbols. We can only explain actions in terms of the meanings that are attributed to them.

We inherit some language and symbols as part of our **culture**. This is the set of attitudes, values, beliefs and meanings which are part of our heritage and define our social identity. Other meanings and values we go on to create ourselves by using language to negotiate with others. In this way we contribute to cultural change and change the way we see the world. Early interactionist work in health drew attention to the ways in which patients seek to make sense of how their lives change following a particular diagnosis or on admission to hospital.

Interactionism takes an **interpretivist** approach. It stresses the importance of understanding or interpreting what things mean to people.

Another such interpretive approach is **phenomenology** – which tries to get inside the subjective perceptions of people to understand fully how they see the world. Alfred Schutz wanted the social sciences to avoid mistakes arising out of hasty attempts to emulate the natural sciences and to stop treating people like inanimate objects. In general, phenomenologists claim that social science *must* take into account the conscious way in which human beings perceive and try to make sense of the world. Thus, like interactionists, phenomenologists not only want to understand how people construct and use meanings, but also strive to understand their experiences.

This is not easy to do. We cannot experience each others' experiences; we can only experience our own. We cannot know how someone else experiences illness or pain, nor can we directly compare someone else's state of health with our own. Language intervenes between us and our individual experiences, so methods have to be constructed to get at those experiences. One of these methods, **ethnomethodology**, analyses the ordinary methods which people use to establish social order and thereby regulate the way in which they relate to each other. Harvey Sacks was an ethnomethodologist who engaged in detailed, meticulous analysis of parts of conversation such as how people greet each other or how they manage to finish a telephone call. The founder of this approach, Harold Garfinkel, used to conduct 'disruption experiments' in which researchers would behave differently in a particular setting in order to lay bare the rules of social order, which are usually unspoken. For example, see what happens when you try to skip your turn in a doctor's waiting room! Such approaches are useful for examining communication and miscommunication in the often brief conversations between doctors and patients or between medical staff.

Structuration theory was developed by Anthony Giddens in the 1980s to draw what was of value from both structuralist and interpretivist perspectives. This theory argues that the actions of individuals and the social structure within which they take place cannot be separated. Individuals do things in the light of others' responses to them and in the awareness of the broader social context within which social interaction occurs. Structure does not physically constrain our actions; it is **immanent**. This means that, although social structures do not have a concrete existence, we behave as if they did and they become a guiding 'presence' which is re-established through our interactions.

Postmodernism has stimulated a great deal of writing on our understanding of the human body and how we deal with it. The work of Michel Foucault (1973) in particular has linked changes in our understanding of illnesses and bodily activities to changes in general social organisation. Postmodernism questions modernist, rationalist assumptions that the world is naturally ordered and can best be understood by rational scientific investigation. Postmodernists see such assumptions as **logocentric**, a way of imposing our method for understanding the world *on* the world. We should not assume too much. The world may not have some underlying order waiting to be discovered. It could be naturally disordered or chaotic, and we are imposing a perspective which enables us to manipulate it.

Postmodernism questions whether an unmediated knowledge of the world is possible. The world is always liable to an interpretation coloured by the assumptions of the viewer. For this reason its focus is upon the 'social construction' of health and illness, primarily through the way in which we talk about these things. What we do with the human body and to it depends upon how we talk about it.

Feminist perspectives examine how more power has been systematically given to men, while women have been made relatively powerless. Most social institutions are **gendered** and the distribution of power within them **contested**; in other words, there is competition for power between men and women. Within the family, education, health, the law and the media, power is distributed unevenly according to gender. Feminist sociologists have aimed at ensuring that both their research methods and the topics they address should not reproduce such disempowerment.

It is argued that women's experiences have been devalued and trivialised, and that they have been represented as subordinate or passive participants and therefore less visible in many social settings. Feminist sociology has therefore contributed to making us more conscious of the multiple interpretations and interests which should be considered in understanding any social institution (Poland 1990).

Some of these theories are easier to use and to understand than others. The **micro-sociological** theories which deal with interpersonal relationships on a small scale are closer to our experiences of being heard and understood by other people. The **macro-sociology** of those theorists interested in large-scale social structures can seem too abstract or too removed from immediate experience. However, their interest in differences in power, in inequality and in the constraints imposed upon us by society is a very real part of our everyday experience. Try the following exercise to see whether you have grasped the central feature of each theory.

Exercise

Each of the theories gives rise to different perspectives on health and illness and what society should do about it. Each of the following statements is *primarily* associated with one of the above theories. Match the theory with the statement.

1. There will always be illness in the world. Illness has a purpose, it fulfils a function in society – but people will only work hard to avoid illness and try to maintain their own and others' health if they get rewarded for it more than someone else who doesn't try to achieve health.

   (Theory = ...)

2. Illness is another one of the consequences of greed – that is, people wanting to have more than others. Health is an unevenly distributed resource and is kept unequal in societies where those who own and control the economic and political system are concerned with the seeking of profit at the expense of everything else – even at the expense of adequate health care for all.

   (Theory = ...)

   cont'd

3. Ideas about health and illness are part of each society's cultural structure. People communicate to each other ideas about their values and their behaviour with regard to health and illness. The ill stay ill because they accept and mutually reinforce the attitudes and practices which got them there in the first place.

(Theory = ...)

4. In reality the world is chaotic, anarchic and unpredictable. The view that the physical world and the natural world has an 'order' or a system to it which we only need to discover is something which goes on in our heads (i.e. in our theories and our ideologies). Health and illness are part of this disorder – they occur randomly, they can happen to anyone, they do not occur systematically.

(Theory = ...)

All these statements are rather crude representations of the theories. They are more likely to match the sorts of thing that people ordinarily say about health and illness. Thus they may entail some mixing of different theories, but they are primarily associated as follows:

1. Functionalism.
2. Marxist conflict theory.
3. Interactionism, with some hints of conflict theory.
4. Postmodernism and/or phenomenology.

Such perspectives are expressed in the ideas about illness and health care that you come across in newspapers and on television, or even views that you hear expressed by your friends and acquaintances. People frequently adopt some mixture of basic theories like these while developing an ideology of their own.

Key questions

To examine the link between theory and ideology consider what would be the consequences of holding such views. In other words, what sorts of policy might be developed by governments holding such views? What sorts of actions might follow in the work of health and social carers if such views were advocated?

The social policy or action consequences of holding such views can range from doing nothing to aiming for the total control of society. For example, from an organic functionalist perspective, a policy of not meddling with the health of social groups might be suggested. They could be allowed to 'evolve naturally' and either grow healthy or die off. On the other hand, a systems approach might support choices about which groups should survive and about social institutions which could be artificially constructed to ensure such an outcome.

Key questions

Which, if any, of the above statements comes closest to your own views? If none, write out a similar statement of your own which does represent your own theory about health and society. Why do some people get ill and not get better, while others do? Why do some people stay healthier than others? Consider what ideology or ideologies you hold. That is, how should our society be organised for the best? Consequently, what would this mean for health care and health policies in general?

A valid theoretical perspective combined with your ideology could provide a focus for action. Problems occur in the move between theory and ideology. Test the accuracy of your views as you read through the rest of this book.

Exercise

Try explaining how the following health-related practices might occur:

1. A group of people are running together. One of them has a bandaged knee and limps. He refuses to cut short his run.

2. A woman is working in a factory. She and her workmates set aside the safety guard on the machinery they are using.

Both situations would sound acceptable if they occurred during wartime – the man running to avoid capture or physical danger, the woman having priorities other than her own physical safety. On the other hand, the man might be afraid to appear weak among a group where macho values of physical strength rule, so he runs on despite his infirmity. Indeed, he may be so obsessed with sport that it dominates his concerns, it being more important to maintain the daily or weekly running regime.

This and the second example may also indicate the importance of belonging to a social group. There may be fear of ridicule for being too fussy, or these may be practices commonly adopted by the group. The pressures of piecework can discourage the use of safety guards. The women's skilled knowledge of the machinery and what risks may be taken is vital. Other pressures could include management requirements for speed, urgency, ignorance of the consequences or legal requirements.

This is the sort of behaviour you need to explain and understand as a health carer.

Conclusion

We will return to each of these theoretical perspectives when we make use of different theories to highlight a particular issue. No single theory can be true; each is more or less useful for a different purpose.

We do not expect you to grasp fully the nature of these perspectives now. You will have a fuller understanding of them and their uses by the end of the book as we explain human social behaviour in all its diversity. We are particularly interested in issues that arise out of the study of society that are relevant for understanding health and illness and how health care is organised and delivered. For this reason we want to emphasise the influence of power and the nature of social inequality throughout the book. Some theoretical perspectives take little notice of relationships of power and oppression while others concentrate on inequality. Ideologies are usually about power – how, when and why to apply it. Power and inequality are central to understanding health care and health policy. Thus, in the next chapter, we will demonstrate the importance of power and control and provide you with the means for conducting your own political analysis.

Further reading

Some introductory sociology texts which explain the theoretical perspectives discussed here in more detail include:

Abercrombie, N. and Warde, A. with Soothill, K., Urry, J. and Walby, S. (1994) *Contemporary British Society*, Oxford: Polity Press.
Giddens, A. (1997) *Sociology* (3rd edn), Cambridge: Polity Press.
O'Donnel, M. (1992) *A New Introduction to Sociology* (3rd edn), Walton-on-Thames: Thomas Nelson & Sons.

Other texts which give a different angle on applying sociology to health are:

Bond, J. & Bond, S. (1993) *Sociology and Health Care* (3rd edn), Edinburgh: Churchill Livingstone.
Scambler, G (ed.) (1991) *Sociology as Applied to Medicine* (3rd edn), London: Baillière Tindall.

The following are medical sociology books which develop in detail the issues which we deal with here:

Fox, N.J. (1993) *Postmodernism, Sociology and Health*, Buckingham: Open University Press.
Murcott, A. (1993) *Health, Disease and Medicine*, Oxford: Blackwell.
Radley, A. (ed.) (1993) *Worlds of Illness: Biographical and Cultural Perspectives on Health and Disease*, London: Routledge.
Stacey, M. (1988) *The Sociology of Health and Healing*, London: Unwin Hyman.

Chapter 2 The Power to Care

One of our main aims is to increase health professionals' awareness of what power they have or can gain access to and to consider how that power might best be used in the interests of their clients. In this chapter we show how the distribution and exercise of power affects the visibility and the value given to different forms of health care work.

The need for power

It may seem odd to suggest that those working in health and care have to understand politics. Your response may even be that you are not interested in politics as you only want to help people. But politics is about power, and anyone who works in a health care system has to learn how to recognise, acquire and use power, both for themselves and for their clients. The gaining and use of power is called **empowerment** and, in this case, it means making it possible to take responsibility for the resources required to do effective care work.

Exercise

Consider this situation:

An anxious, partly clothed patient has been kept waiting in a draughty corridor long after their due appointment time.

Who had the power to make them wait so long and in such a setting?

cont'd

> What power will the patient have to do anything about it?
> How can the patient become empowered?

You can see from the questions and your answers that this is a political situation. It involves some people having control over others and some not even having control over their own situation.

Politics is not only about how politicians and government do their work; it is found anywhere in society – in social clubs, in families or in work. Social relationships in families and workplaces are political because they are based on differences in power. Politics goes on in any situation where people struggle to use power. To secure health goals or ensure adequate services for dealing with poor health, you have to handle disagreements about services and treatment. This means acting politically with managers, administrators, colleagues and clients.

Power can be defined as the ability of individuals or groups to get others to do what they want them to do, even when those others do not want to do it. Exercising power can take a variety of forms from using gentle persuasion to physical force.

Authority is a form of power which is seen as legitimate. It is the form of power most frequently used by the health care professional with a client. For example, you would not usually undress for most people merely because they ask you to. When a doctor during a consultation asks you to undress, you do so because you recognise their authority. According to Max Weber (1925), we comply with those in authority because we see them as having either:

- a **legal** right to tell people what do;
- **traditional** rights to power – they are obeyed because they always have been;

or

- **charisma** – personal characteristics which enable them to persuade others.

In any real-life situation, the authority applied in practice may be a mixture of these three main types.

Key questions

What forms of authority are being used when:

- you receive a letter from the council asking you to pay your council tax;
- your parents ask you to do something;
- someone you admire or respect asks a favour?

You might respect some individual members of local government but, on the whole, when you pay local taxes it is because of your legal/rational relationship with them – you have made a contract to that effect. Parents might be respected owing to traditional authority, although you might respect them individually to such an extent that you see them as charismatic. The favour for someone you admire seems solely done for their charismatic authority.

Political resources

In addition to authority, your having the power to persuade other people to behave in a particular way or to hold particular views will depend on whether or not you have the means to influence them. The means of influence, persuasion or force are **political resources**. Power is applied by offering, using or withholding such resources.

Exercise

Use the following checklist of resources to test the extent of your own power.

Ask a colleague which resources they think that you possess – you may be surprised!

RESOURCES CHECKLIST

	A lot	A little	None at all
Economic resources:			
money	____	____	____
property	____	____	____
shares	____	____	____
Personal resources:			
the ability to work (labour power)	____	____	____
physical strength	____	____	____
physical attractiveness	____	____	____
craft/artistic skills	____	____	____
communication skills	____	____	____
social standing (prestige)	____	____	____
leadership qualities	____	____	____
sexual favours	____	____	____
administrative skills	____	____	____
knowledge	____	____	____
the ability to retrieve information (find things out)	____	____	____
Collective resources:			
organisational backing	____	____	____
access to mass media	____	____	____
social (friendship) networks	____	____	____
family connections	____	____	____

cont'd

State:

access to the law	____	____	____
police	____	____	____
military force	____	____	____
control over secret information	____	____	____

Now consider – would you have more or less of these resources:

... among your family?	More ____	or Less ____
... in educational settings?	More ____	or Less ____
... in your sports/leisure club?	More ____	or Less ____
... as a care professional?	More ____	or Less ____
... as a patient ?	More ____	or Less ____

Your responses to these questions show that **power is not a fixed resource**. It is **relative** to the setting in which it operates. For example, some people have more power in their paid work than they do in their household. Most of us have more power at home, in our leisure or recreational activities than anywhere else, perhaps making them more enjoyable. Ask yourself, in those settings in which you have more power, what extra resources do you have? In those settings in which you have less power, what resources do you have less of?

Exercise

Using the resource list above, try analysing the following situation politically:

A younger member of your family consumes a nutritionally poor diet.

You try to influence them to improve their diet.

To do this, list the resources you have and those of your younger relative, explain the power differentials involved and discuss the likely outcomes to the situation.

Age differentials can give rise to power differentials. For example, children have less power since they often lack resources of physical strength, knowledge, information and money. Oddly enough, this can change in old age – children may have more strength and information than their grandparents. However, all of these power differentials can be complicated by membership of the same family and the authority relationships involved. No matter how good the knowledge and information you hold, if a younger person has no respect for your authority, you will not be listened to.

People can enhance their power by acting in different settings and by attempting to acquire more of the resources which give them power. Which resources listed above can you most easily acquire? There are usually constraints on quickly gaining economic or material resources, but all of us can do a lot more than we realise to gain communication skills and knowledge, and to make use of social networks. In reading this book you are enhancing your power by increasing your knowledge and improving your communication skills.

Similarly, we can gain power by using *collective* resources. There is strength in numbers through joining trades unions, professional associations or community groups. The backing of such organisations can help us to persuade other people. Some political resources can be spent up when they are used. We lose physical energy in using *force* and, if we use up *wealth*, we will have less at our disposal to use as a resource in the future. Other resources can actually grow the more they are used. Skills such as *knowledge* and *communication* improve with practice. The more practised you are at operating politically, the more effectiveness and credibility you will gain in caring for people.

The distribution of power

The approach we suggest here is what Dahl (1984) calls 'pluralist political analysis'. It shows how all of us have some power, even though some people have much more than others. Few people have no power at all.

Exercise

Make a list of the sorts of people who possess a lot of these political resources and make a similar list of others who possess very little.

Those with a lot of   **Those with little power**
power/resources

Go back to these lists as you read through the book and see whether you want to make changes to them.

Political resources are unevenly distributed. Throughout society, within local communities and within the family, some individuals have more power than others. In our lists those with more power include monarchs, dictators, politicians, doctors, managers, teachers and men; those with less power include women, housewives, the unemployed and senior citizens.

Key questions

You can analyse this in more detail by answering the following questions:

● Who holds the remote control unit when the family are watching television?

● Who is the first to answer the telephone?

● Who knows what state the family finances are in?

● Who does the shopping?

● Who makes the decisions about the expensive purchases for the household?

What matters, of course, is how important such decisions are for the lives of family members. **Decision-making** is a significant act of power, and while some people may appear to have a lot of power they may be unable to take key decisions. Similarly, some people appear to have very little power in general but can take decisions which may significantly influence someone's life. For example, the person behind the counter in a social security office may have little power in general terms, and they may not take the decisions about who is entitled to how much money, but they have the power to interpret those decisions in order to allocate the available finance.

However, as Lukes (1974) has pointed out, people do not always find themselves in situations in which decisions can be made. Indeed, a powerful individual may be someone who sets up a situation to prevent decision-making or where there is only a choice between unfavoured options. Thus putting more money into health care seems an unlikely option in the contemporary climate, so we are left with 'deciding' how to spend the little we have. It may even be the case that a group is so powerful that allowing others to share in decision-making threatens the dominant ideology. Thus it took many years for women to have a say in political decision-making.

Simply looking at who commands most resources can tell us who possesses most power. It is important to ask why resources are distributed unevenly and why some people can take certain decisions whereas others cannot. Such questions will aid your understanding of the consequences of an uneven distribution of power in the provision of health and caring services.

Power in caring

> Excellence requires commitment and involvement, but it also requires power. (Benner 1984: 207)

Caring means taking responsibility for people. To fulfil that responsibility requires power. If, for example, an elderly or infirm person needs food, the carer has to know how to get it and how to give it. Responsibility without power would lead to ineffective caring. Traditionally, the qualities appropriate to a caring role have been linked to subservience and self-sacrifice and have therefore been a source of powerlessness. In hierarchies which involve competition, control and domination, masculine forms of power have been viewed as more important. This is partly how society devalues women, women's work and, as a consequence, much of health care. This view implies that women and carers will only gain power if they adopt male perspectives on power.

Because the political resources entailed in caring have not been traditionally accorded a high status in power hierarchies, that is no reason to underestimate them. Instead, they should be recognised and understood. It is clear that health care professionals 'can have enormous power over how a patient will spend their first or last hours on earth' (Benner 1984: 216). What could be more powerful in the life of an individual?

Patricia Benner (1984) has listed the qualities of power associated with caring as follows:

1. **Transformative power** – enabling clients to hold a new perspective on their illness, their treatment and life in general.

2. **Integrative caring** – enabling the individual to reintegrate into their social world, either in convalescence or in dealing with permanent disability.

3. **Advocacy** – translating medical jargon and overcoming the patient's anxieties.

4. **Healing power** – mobilising hope, interpreting the situation and assisting in the use of social, emotional and spiritual support.

5. **Affirmative power** – commitment to and involvement in a caring relationship.

6. **Problem-solving** – expertise in perceiving the likely causes and consequences of a problem.

Benner applies these qualities to nursing, but they apply to all health care roles.

Exercise

Look at how you could apply the resources listed above and your caring power in the following situation:

You are the son or daughter of a parent who smokes.

You attempt to convince them to stop.

Once more explain the power differentials involved and discuss the likely outcomes to the situation.

Again there is an age differential. Knowledge and information differences between you and your parent are likely, but their assumed authority and the addictive hold that a smoking habit has on people is difficult to challenge. It is possible that your caring power – your belief that smoking is bad for their health combined with your care for their health – could help to swing the balance of power in your favour.

The power of patients

Patients have less power than health professionals, partly because of the vulnerabilities they suffer as a consequence of their illness and partly because they are in unfamiliar territory when seeking treatment. Even experienced health professionals perceive a loss of power when they find themselves as patients.

By gaining access to the appropriate resources they can enhance their power in the clinical situation. As Nagler (1993) shows even long-term disabled patients can acquire resources to redress their political inequality. Such 'patient power' depends upon the existence of patients' rights groups and on improved knowledge and information about illness complaints and about treatment procedures. Legal support for consumer choice can enhance patients' power.

The power of health care professionals

In addition to the caring power outlined above, health professionals also have a certain amount of authority in their relationships with clients:

- **Legal** – the state permits them to do things to and for their clients that other people are not legitimately entitled to do. Lawler (1991) shows how such authority is vital to gain access to the body and to conduct physically invasive procedures.
- **Traditional** – many patients do as they are told by health professionals because they have always done so.
- **Charismatic** – health care professionals are held in high esteem in the community at large. Doctors' views are

respected owing to their assumed knowledge and expertise.
All health care professionals are respected for their
knowledge about illness and their commitment to caring.

These forms of authority are backed up by the assumption that
health care professionals operate more in the interests of their
clients than themselves. This has made it difficult for them to
apply a resource available to many other workers: the right to
withdraw labour and go on strike. Until recently, health care
professionals have had little access to those material and
economic resources which determine the conditions under which
they work and provide services.

What power will they need to do their job properly in future?

One of the key changes taking place in caring services in the UK is
devolution – a move from centralised planning to a more local
control of scarce health care resources. These changes have
included:

- the establishment of independent Trust status for hospitals;
- fundholding in general practice;
- community care;
- the growing use of informal, family and home carers;
- a shortage of institutional provision.

Central government fixes the constraints within which the new
health and care system has to operate. Once again it is important
to ask 'Who actually makes the key decisions about resources?' It
is likely that such resources will become increasingly limited and
subject to competition.

These changes are typical of health care throughout the world.
As the nature of health and social care systems change health care
professionals have to consider and develop their political
resources to do their job effectively. Those working lower down
the hierarchy have to take on more managerial responsibilities,
but they may not be *given* more power to obtain or to control
resources. They will acquire new kinds of authority in the
community as they enhance their skills in needs assessment, in

the use of technical equipment and in prescribing treatment. Behind these changes is an emphasis on the **health service user as a consumer**. This raises the importance of client advocacy, professional responsibility and accountability as political resources.

Fundamentally, professionals will have to enhance their knowledge base and their information retrieval skills, and to do so from a multidisciplinary perspective. They will need more technical knowledge and communication skills, and an improved understanding of psycho-social needs. They will also need knowledge of the groups within the community – their culture, ethnicity and family, leisure and work patterns. These are all areas in which a sociological perspective is vital.

What are the limits on the redistribution of power?

Health care professionals will have to redefine their place within a changing occupational structure. It will be difficult to overcome traditional power hierarchies and to develop new practices for standing up to those groups which have traditionally wielded power. Forms of clothing and uniforms, for example, have been traditional markers or signifiers of authority in the medical hierarchy. They make much less sense within the new occupational structure.

Constraints on the goals of health care will have to be confronted. Managers and administrators who control resources may not necessarily agree with health care practitioners on identifying and measuring effective patient care or treatment outcomes. Managers are used to **measurable performance indicators** or ways in which to demonstrate how far organisational goals are achieved. Caring is particularly hard to quantify and measure. Cost–benefit analyses of the resources for health and caring are done more in the interest of wider society than in the interests of an individual client. Bureaucrats, doctors and other health carers may all have different goals.

Collecting evidence from research is important for developing and exercising knowledge which will give weight to an argument. Resources will always remain a limiting factor but, with accurate information and the skills to communicate it, health professionals will be more able to argue for policies to accomplish their own primary goals.

Conclusion: Political empowerment

Empowerment is not only about giving resources to people who appear not to have them; those who hold resources are usually unwilling to give them up. Empowerment entails encouraging people to recognise what resources they have, which ones can be used to gain more and, ultimately, which ones will help them to achieve their goals as health professional or client.

Traditionally, health carers have tended to be politically apathetic. As a modern health professional you must be able to reflect on and assess your work situation, to decide upon what actions are needed given your assessment and then to judge how best to implement those decisions. Political awareness requires that you analyse a situation, set goals and engage in tactics that will achieve your objectives. Successful caring requires that health professionals take key roles in the management of change to accomplish cherished goals and to maintain values in caring. This means operating politically.

Key questions

Use the following questions to check your understanding of the issues covered in this chapter. Consider your own responses and discuss them with others:

- What kinds of authority do health care professionals have?
- What extra political resources are needed for effective health care work?
- How can health care professionals use their power to enhance their effectiveness?
- Why should health professionals be more politically aware?

We will return to the gaining and use of political resources in subsequent chapters, but first, in Chapter 3, we will show how our understanding of caring relationships is entrenched in the process by which we learn to become a fully fledged member of society. This, too, is a 'power-full' experience.

Further reading

Benner, P. (1984) 'Excellence and power in clinical nursing practice', Chapter 14, pp. 207–20 in Benner, P. *From Novice to Expert: Excellence and Power in Clinical Nursing Practice*, California: Addison-Wesley.
A readable, competent political analysis of the health carer's role.

Brandon, D. (1991) *Direct Power: A Handbook on Service Brokerage*, Preston: Tao Publications.
Useful for understanding emerging power relationships in health and social care provision.

Hart, N. (1985) *The Sociology of Health and Medicine*, Ormskirk: Causeway Press, Chapters 3, 6 and 7.
Easy to read on power in health systems.

Serving, R. (1996) *Theorising Empowerment: Individual Power and Community Care*, Bristol: The Policy Press.
Looks further at most of the issues raised in this chapter.

Turner, B.S. (1987) *Medical Power and Social Knowledge*, London: Sage.
Frames all medical sociology in terms of the understanding of power relationships.

Chapter 3 Learning to Care: A Lifetime of Socialisation

Throughout life we learn how to become members of different kinds of group, ranging from family groups, through groups of friends, to school and work groups. We learn each group's language, its values and its practices. We learn how to work and play in groups. In the company of other people our own identity emerges and we learn further how to interact with others.

We have different learning experiences of health care depending upon whether or not we become patients or health care professionals. Many professionals tell of the change in perspective they gain from having to be a patient. This shows that we continue to learn about what it is to become a member of a group and how to behave appropriately in different settings. Our power grows as we gain insider knowledge, but may be limited by broader constraints on us such as our age, gender, skills and wealth. There are many imbalances in care relationships based on our access to resources.

> **Exercise**
>
> Write down anything you noticed about the most recent group you joined. How were you treated as a 'new member'? What stood out for you about the kind of language used? How do members address one another? How did you learn or are you learning the kinds of attitudes and behaviour that are deemed appropriate in the group?

Socialisation

Human behaviour is influenced partly by factors from our biological **nature** and partly by factors from our culture – how we are **nurtured**. As children we begin a lifelong process of learning about who we are and how we may act within society. This process is called **socialisation** and takes place when we experience taking part in various groups and organisations. Typically these groups include families and home environments, schools, peer groups and leisure groups.

As we mature we join many other kinds of group, including work organisations and occupational and professional groups. Becoming a member of any group means learning about that group's values, understandings and rules of behaviour. When passing on such knowledge, groups act as **agencies of socialisation**. In complex industrialised societies adults are expected to have undergone a variety of socialisation experiences.

Childhood is widely seen as a stage in our lives when we are constantly learning. We are told about who we are and how to act in situations and settings that are new to us. However, learning how to act in different groups is a process which is lifelong rather than simply limited to the **primary socialisation** of childhood. For example, becoming members of health care professions, with specialist knowledge of health and caring services, calls for specialist training and some **secondary socialisation** which comes with new knowledge, values and standards. It also requires an appreciation of the diversity of socialisation experiences of clients and other carers.

There are competing theoretical perspectives on socialisation. **Functionalists** stress that individuals acquire the commonly accepted knowledge which they need to play their part within the system. This suggests that individuals who lack vital knowledge will find themselves marginalised on attempting to join some groups or may behave inappropriately in some social settings. The experience of children with disabilities who have spent long periods in large institutions supports such a view. It is difficult for them to rejoin outside groups. In the same way patients being admitted to hospital, or medical students working on wards for the first time, need to learn how to behave.

Other perspectives see socialisation as a two-way process. **Interactionists** do not see it as cultural programming but as the building of shared understandings between people. This entails becoming aware that people vary in their values and **norms** – the prescriptions for how they ought to behave. Co-operation is impossible without negotiation. For example, Becker (1961) has shown how medical students do not accept new medical knowledge in an undiscriminating way. They match what they are told with what they see happening. They ignore instructions which do not fit, or which create conflict, choosing instead actions which appear reasonable and expedient. In the same way Melia (1987) shows how student nurses are not just 'empty vessels to be filled' but participate actively in the selection of norms, values and attitudes to shape their socialisation according to their own goals.

Peer groups of our own age and background are important in shaping our identity, expectations and activities. We also gain images and information about the social world and our place in it from the mass media. **Rites of passage** mark our arrival in the world, the transition from childhood to adulthood and various changes in adult status. Some of these – such as smoking, drinking alcohol and sex – may be problematic if taken up when very young. There may be tensions between youth and adult cultures. Understanding these issues is important for health professionals in developing health education and understanding health care issues relating to children and young people.

Given the divisions between the resources, values and activities of different social groups, the socialisation experiences available through them provide key pointers to potential inequalities between individuals. Childhood experiences are not the same for everyone. People have highly diverse experiences among their families and in school. This is called **social differentiation** and suggests why our life, educational and health chances vary widely.

An example of **social differentiation through socialisation** is that of gender. Rubin *et al.* (1974) have shown that, even when there are few overt physical differences between babies, there is evidence that parents describe them differently according to gender: girls as smaller, softer and less attentive, boys as stronger, more alert and better co-ordinated. Smith and Lloyd (1978) describe how adults are more likely to encourage boys to take part in physical activities and to offer them trucks or blocks as toys than girls, who would be offered dolls. Fagot (1984) documents how parents show more approval when children behave appropriately to their sex and react negatively otherwise, although 'tomboys' are more tolerated than 'cissies'. This fostering of gender differences is subtly reinforced in school: girls are rewarded more than boys for silence, neatness and conformity. Peer group socialisation further shapes gender identity as friendship groups are usually single sex.

Media images sustain **gender stereotyping**. Males are depicted as adventurous, authoritative, independent and strong. Females are confined to indoor activities in domestic, passive or subordinate roles. Hospital dramas, for example, reinforce stereotyping by showing emotional, subordinate female nurses looking up to decisive male doctors and caring for male patients with injuries brought about by daring behaviour. Schooling and media agencies of socialisation have changed to respond to feminist research and campaigning by professional organisations. Diversity in learning activities is now available to both sexes, and there are images of women in more active and authoritative positions.

Exercise

List the kinds of gender socialisation that you have experienced. What attitudes and behaviour were expected of you because of your gender? Are there any differences in gender expectations between the different groups you belong to?

Socialisation is a complex interactive process through which an individual develops socially, emotionally, intellectually and behaviourally. Experiences with socialisation agencies are mediated through individual biographical events and broader social differences such as class, ethnicity and gender. These influence how individuals acquire and develop skills, knowledge, attitudes, values, beliefs and interests. We deal with each of these influences in more detail in following chapters.

Play and games

Socialisation is accomplished in most societies through play. Playing appears to be an entirely free activity since it is most obvious in the world of children. However, even from a very early age, play is structured, often around interactions with others. It offers a way to practise being in a group without the serious consequences that doing the activity 'for real' would have. Adults play for the same reasons as children.

Play may be exploratory, physical, creative, imaginative, co-operative and problem-solving. As children grow older the complexity of the forms of play in which they can engage develops from **solitary**, through **parallel** (where they do activities similar to those of another child but without sharing play), to **interactive** (where the play is based on shared action).

During **games**, participants carefully clarify and insist on the **rules** to be observed while maintaining distinctions between play and reality. Rules are negotiated or controlled according to the power of various participants. Play contains elements of ritual such as chanting, or clapping and repetitive behaviour. Games require regularised turn-taking. These are ways to learn the interactive skills needed successfully to take part in social life, to learn group behaviour and to take on **social roles**, ways of 'being' in the group.

As children get older their play is less repetitious or stylised. Bearing the consequences of rule-breaking or exclusions in play can also prepare for encounters with power and point to the limits on power. Adult playing allows temporary escape from the serious business of life but also sets the boundaries to work and leisure relationships. Adult games are also bound by rules.

Exercise

Observe examples of play and games for children of at least two different ages or social groups. Notice the ways in which play is 'serious' and 'rule-governed' rather than a completely free activity. What social skills are learned in these ways?

How does play involving 'make believe' differ from 'real life' adult role-taking?

cont'd

What similar kinds of social knowledge were gained in the play you observed?

What are the needs of children whose access to play is restricted by their own illness or disability, or by the illness or disability of significant adults in their lives?

In what ways might children with special learning needs have found it difficult to take part in the play activity which you observed? How may they have been helped to participate?

It is easy to see how the exclusion of ill or disabled children from normal play has consequences for other areas of their social learning, in terms of their skills and sense of power and control. Facilitating such participation needs attention to whether extra time, explanation of rules or other kinds of preparation can be provided by a helper. Sometimes children within a family, community or school learn how to provide such help since they pay closer attention to games and play than do adults.

Social identity

Through socialisation and in our relationships with other people we take on **social roles**. This means that we 'act' in a certain way in social situations. You might say that you never act differently, that you always try to be 'true to yourself', but have you ever been nice to someone when they were not being nice to you? Have you ever disliked someone but tried not to show it? That sort of behaviour is something that health care professionals often have to do with their clients, that is, **playing a role**. It may be a crucial element in caring for someone. It is not that we are being false, but we recognise that we sometimes have to control ourselves and others through role play.

Sometimes we do these things self-consciously, with a heightened awareness of what we are doing. At other times our role behaviour becomes such a habit that we are unconscious of it. Being a son or daughter, a mother or father, a sister or brother, is not something we have to think about. Unlike family and gender roles, professional role playing requires us to think clearly about what we are doing and how others see us. It is possible to improve professional skills by being able to analyse such roles.

Concepts of self and personal identity

Most individuals have an awareness of their individuality. We all have a concept of **self**, a unique identity which singles us out from others. This poses a sociological problem: in what ways do these unique individuals behave separately and still create patterns in society?

Much of the work of the psychiatrist R.D. Laing (1967, 1969, 1971) was based on the idea that we have 'real' and 'false' selves – the real 'us' and the selves we put up for public presentation. He pointed out that we can never directly experience any one else's experiences. To know what someone else knows depends upon **reciprocating cognition**. This means us having a sense of their experiences and them having a sense of ours. The only way in which we come to an awareness of what someone else is going through is by communicating with them. However, human communication is so complicated by ambiguity, error and contradiction that misunderstandings about our true experiences can arise. For example, Baron-Cohen (1995) suggests that autistic children lack the ability to 'read the minds' of others, that is, understanding situations from another person's point of view.

Key questions

- How do you view your 'self'?
- Is there an inner core self which is only known to you?
- Do you believe that anyone really knows you?
- If they do, what is it that they know?

These are philosophical and spiritual questions to which there is no easy answer. It is difficult to separate our beliefs from our experiences and from the logical problems which such questions pose. What is interesting is the variety of responses to these questions.

Social scientists generally agree that we are not born with a self-concept. It develops over time, emerging out of our interaction with the physical and social environment. It can be argued that individual development involves gradually mastering the social environment, or that the social environment gradually imposes itself on the individual. In both cases there is some reciprocal adaptation of the individual with the environment. Our sense of 'being' depends on the material and social objects to which we relate. The sense of a unique self or identity depends upon the environment in which we operate and develop.

The concept of role

The problem is that we never relate *directly* to the people and things around us. The relationship between our self and the environment is mediated by the part we are playing in any specific situation. This might depend on the job we do there or the people we are with or, more probably, a combination of both. This 'part we are playing' is what is meant by the term **social role**. A role develops out of how we are expected to behave in social situations and how we actually behave. We think, feel and act largely in terms of our conception of the role we are in at any given time.

It is because social roles exist at the intersection between the individual and society that some sociologists suggest that one can never perceive an individual's true self since, in any given social situation, we only observe an individual through the role they are playing at the time.

Key questions

- Do you agree with this?
- Given what you thought about your 'self' earlier, do you see it as accessible?
- Can anyone get to the 'real you', separate from the part you are playing in a role?

Our sense of personal identity is very different from our concept of our role. Our concept of self distinguishes us from other humans. It transcends the many roles we play in that we can take our sense of self with us to all the situations in which we find ourselves, but other unique selves could just as easily play the same role we do. Thus, given your absence for a period of time, someone else could take on your professional role.

Role awareness is based upon several layers of conceptualisation. Figure 3.1 clarifies these layers diagrammatically. In any specific social situation:

a   the individual has a conception of their role;

b   other people in that situation have a conception of the role;

c   the individual has an idea that others hold a conception of their role.

The people who interact with the individual are referred to as **significant others** since their role conceptions and their behaviour in relation to the individual have a significant influence on how the individual plays the role. However, since roles exist independently of the individual, other people in society have views about how people ought to behave in specific situations.

This means we have to bring in **d** – the **generalised other**. This comprises the larger demands of the social structure: rules, laws and general social expectations. Such general expectations of the role are more formally prescribed and expected to hold for most situations. Where a role is related to an organisation, this layer comprises that organisation's regulations for behaviour. The significant others use this generalised other as a frame of reference for the correct role behaviour which they expect from the individual. Then, at layer **e**, the individual has an awareness of these larger social expectations and acts in light of them.

So far we have referred only to **expectations** about how roles ought to be played. Such abstract notions have to be related to the actual behaviour itself – layer **f** – our **role performance**. The way in which we and others enact roles can then be observed.

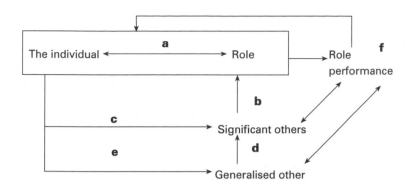

Figure 3.1   Levels of awareness in the role concept

Our subsequent role expectations can then be constructed on the basis of our observations and experience of repeated role performances. Estimations of whether or not the correct role has been adopted or the role has been 'played' correctly are based on prior experiences of the performance of a role and on what society tells us to expect. It is here that socialisation agencies have a key part to play. The family, the media and educational institutions all provide us with ideas about how to play a role even before we find ourselves in the situation.

By understanding these different layers of awareness we can analyse the components of each of the many roles that we play. Such analysis can focus attention on how co-operation between individuals is built upon social bargains. In order to co-operate with one another we need to build expectations about how people are likely to behave when we meet them. We have **mutual expectations** about how we expect each other to behave. Co-operation and trust between individuals, which is essential to social order, depends on role expectations being fulfilled in role performances.

Exercise

This analysis can be applied to any of the roles we play. Look at the roles you play: son or daughter, brother or sister, parent, child, nurse, doctor, midwife, friend, carer. What are your expectations of the role? How do others expect you to play it? What are the generalised expectations within society about the role? How far does your performance of the role match these expectations? How will those expectations change in light of your performance?

Key questions

Another way of highlighting role expectations and performance is to remember the first time you played a particular role. Remember the first time you had an alcoholic drink, made love or provided personal care.

- How did you know what to do?

- Did your performance match your expectations?

- Did others' performance match your expectations?

- How do you know whether you fulfilled or altered others' expectations?

Different theoretical views

There are varying theoretical perspectives on the concept of social role. The functionalist view stresses the importance of levels **d** and **e** in Figure 3.1, arguing that each role player is constrained to conform to the **structured expectations** of society. The interactionist perspective emphasises the **b** and **c** components of Figure 3.1, suggesting that the role-player's behaviour has to do with the **social process** of negotiating expectations between the individual and significant others.

The functionalist view sees roles as fixed by the social structure rather than by the individuals playing them. Role expectations are seen as becoming institutionalised over time as a result of repeat performances. Individuals continue to play roles in a similar way because law, custom, social conventions and habit lead them to absorb the **normative structure** of society. Playing roles confirms the perceived reality of law and custom. Functionalists argue that internalising role expectations is one of the significant formative processes of human life. In taking on roles an individual surrenders their individuality.

Interactionists see roles in a less rigid way. They argue that a role is constantly being redefined and modified by the individual. They suggest that a role concept is a common-sense tool for understanding or interpreting, rather than simply constraining, human behaviour. We all use the 'idea' of a role to confer meaning to action. Interactionists acknowledge that how a role is defined depends on shared values and meanings within a given group.

Role concepts help us to prepare for a range of responses for different situations. Expectations are confirmed or denied. Using words, gestures and behaviour we negotiate with certain people an appropriate role relationship which can become relatively stabilised – but only with those people and in that sort of situation. The next time we find ourselves with others we begin again, with a tentative concept of the appropriate role to adopt. From an interactionist point of view social structures become a framework rather than a determinant of social action, and roles are not fixed. Instead, they can be changed in their performance. This emphasises social negotiation rather than constraint. It sounds more complex than it is. Most of us negotiate all the time without much thought, especially if we have acquired the relevant social skills to recognise what other people expect of us. We can then make our own rapid decisions about how to adjust our role behaviour accordingly.

Exercise

Look at the role which you analysed above. Which aspects of the role do you have some freedom in playing and which do you feel you could not change even if you wanted to?

It helps to see social roles as partly structured and partly negotiable. Understanding the distinctions within the role concept may help in explaining the problems and difficulties arising out of people's attempts to perform their roles. The most immediate value of such an analysis can be seen in the way in which conflicts within and between roles can arise.

Role conflict

Conflict within a role (**intra-role conflict**) arises when there is a dysjunction between the individual's role expectations and the expectations of others in the role relationship. This entails a dysjunction between layers **a** and **b** in Figure 3.1. An example of this is when you, as a health professional, have to give a client bad news. You may wish to be honest and accurate; the client may not want to hear bad news. You have to make an adjustment between the client's expectations about your news and your own judgement about what you can say. You may realise the conflicting expectations during interaction with the client (via level **c** in Figure 3.1) and resolve the conflict by adjusting your role performance accordingly. Such conflict may be intensified when none of the participants in the role relationship is aware of the others' expectations, and it is then that mistakes in giving bad news are made. Role conflict may be experienced as a very real personal dilemma.

The most common form of role conflict occurs between roles (**inter-role conflict**) and arises out of the fact that each individual plays many roles. A female, for example, may be mother, daughter, wife, shop assistant, passenger, patient, friend and so on. Acting on the expectations associated with any one of these roles may conflict with the expectations associated with any of the other roles. For example, the family physician may use humour inappropriately during a clinical consultation with a patient who is also a close neighbour. The conflict for the doctor is between the roles of neighbour and clinician.

This analysis also aids our understanding of **role distance**. This occurs when we, as ordinary members of society, stand back from the entire role-playing situation and adopt a detached awareness of its structure. We do this with varying levels of awareness. It appears more likely to happen in the early stages of performing a role or when leaving it. Teachers have commented to us that they remember their self-consciousness of the teacher role when they started lecturing. The same thing happens to those new to the student role or to the professional role.

Sick role

Sociologists have used the concept of role to understand the behaviour and expectations of people when they are ill. Illness disturbs the normal functioning of the individual, so it has social and psychological, as well as biological, consequences. A distinction is drawn between the **illness** which is perceived by the sufferer, the **disease** which is identified by the doctor, and **sickness**, which is culturally defined as a legitimate social role.

Illness is disturbing to the individual and to society because it interferes with social roles. It is managed by establishing a set of role relationships around the ill person – the **sick role**. Telles and Pollack (1981) point out recognised role stages in the process of being ill. Progress through these stages is as much dependent on psychological and social (**psycho-social**) factors as it is on physiological, biochemical or anatomical factors. As a social process it is subject to change and differs between individuals and communities. Identifying such a process means that we can show that people do not simply seek medical attention because they are ill or experiencing pain. People have symptoms for which they do not seek attention, and there are distinct non-physiological triggers to the decision to seek medical aid. Each stage in the process is partly negotiated with others and partly a consequence of the individual's reflections. Pain is not always the first sign that there is a problem; it may not even be present. At other times pain may be the only indicator that there is a problem.

Recognition of a problem

This involves feeling 'different' in some way or a changed perception of 'normal' health standards. Some standards of health are seen as more significant than others. A measurable departure from physiological standards such as temperature and blood pressure justifies feeling different. Health and illness are measured, managed and experienced in terms of feelings. We assume that feelings are determined by physiological states. A doctor's confirmation legitimises these feelings. This is why it is so problematic when we feel ill and the doctor 'can find nothing wrong'.

Perception of impairment

The severity of impairment can vary widely. There are both physical and psycho-social consequences. Normal social relationships can be impaired, as can normal occupational tasks. Often the more severe the physical impairment, the greater the psycho-social impairment. However, some people with severe physical impairments establish social routines which allow for their disabilities. For them social impairment is only caused by new developments in their disorder which prevent them from carrying on their routines.

The perception of how severe the impairment is may depend on interactions with others. Others may verify or deny that the person is ill. They will indicate which kinds and amounts of feeling are acceptable and which can be legitimately complained about. The sick person may find ways to demonstrate the validity of their feelings. They may groan or grimace or faint, bleed or vomit, but others may still doubt the authenticity of the symptoms. Nurses make relative judgements about which patients are genuinely in pain and which are 'acting up'. Some of these symptoms can be regarded as legitimate markers of illness, so the ultimate official legitimator of illness, the doctor, can be called in at this point.

Seeking help

Depending on the nature of the problem, help-seeking ranges from looking for information about the problem, self-help, asking a friend and consulting the local pharmacist to visiting a doctor. Social factors again intervene. Some people suffer a condition for a long time, feeling they cannot afford the time off. Others may malinger, using the smallest problem as an excuse. Similarly, family obligations and responsibilities intervene in the decision to seek help. What also happens at this stage is what Zola (1973) called a **'temporalising of symptomatology'** – setting a time limit on symptoms before help is sought.

Both the extent and the nature of the help sought is subject to psycho-social influences. For example, Jehovah's Witnesses refuse blood transfusions on religious grounds. Some people prefer 'natural' treatments rather than 'artificial' ones like drugs or surgery. In this stage we see more directly the influence of political, economic and moral questions. Thus decisions about surgical priorities, kidney machines, hospital beds and the number of trained physicians are dependent not just on physiological, but also on socially structured criteria. Yet these will determine the help which can be sought.

Exercise

Using the role concept and the 'stages' of illness approach, analyse your own experiences of illness or the experiences of others which you have observed. Did you or they go through each of these stages? What sorts of thing determined entry to and exit from the sick role? Did you or they enter the patient role? What determined whether you (or they) cared for yourself or were cared for by others?

A determining factor in all these stages is the severity of the condition, but diagnosis, treatment and prognosis do not take place in a social vacuum. For the same condition different diagnoses, treatment and prognoses can result depending upon the doctor's view of how a patient may react to the information about the condition, the patient's view of what is acceptable and, ultimately, the resources available.

Expectations of the sick role

Parsons' (1951) view of the sick role has been criticised for being too 'functionalist' in perspective. Nonetheless, he does identify the major expectations commonly linked to the sick role:

1. Depending upon the nature and severity of the illness normal role responsibilities are relaxed. We are not expected to do things we normally do.

2. The sick are assumed not to be responsible for whether or not they get better.

3. However, because illness is defined as undesirable, there is an obligation on the individual to try to get well and exit the role as soon as possible.

4. There is an obligation to seek technically competent help. If we are not getting better naturally or with informal help, obligations (2) and (3) require us to try to do as much about it as we can.

This last stage leads us into the **patient role**, in which the above obligations and expectations are strenuously asserted. Once someone becomes a patient a special category of sick role is established. Relations between the individual and their carer are formalised. Once again decisions to seek medical aid are not solely related to the physical nature and causes of the illness. They are connected to social, psychological and even economic pressures. There may be further temporalising of the symptomatology. Can you afford to pay for the prescription or spare the time to be ill?

Most people do not actively seek the sick role, and it is assumed to be only temporary. Any contravention of these expectations may lead to a view of the individual as somehow 'deviant'. Thus those actively seeking the role range from the hypochondriac to someone suffering from Munchausen's syndrome in which a physically healthy individual seeks surgical intervention. Those who are physically or mentally disabled or even terminally ill may be legitimately allowed a permanent sick role. To some extent the expectations on the individual are the same as for other sick roles. They are expected to seek technical help and not to want to remain in that condition. However, the permanence of the condition will remove blame from the individual for not actively seeking to get better.

It is vital to remember that the sick role is rarely the *only* role that a person plays – it need not be entirely comprehensive or pervasive. Like all the other roles we play it is one among many. The patient is also a father or mother, husband or wife, son or daughter, a teacher, student, friend and so on. Of course, there are times when it will become a dominant role, overriding all other concerns. This usually happens when patients are so incapacitated that they are prevented from taking on any other roles.

Another special feature of the sick role is that it is a private and individual experience. Apart from more chronic conditions, there tends to be little opportunity to share in a subculture. However, the more recent growth of self-help groups has helped in sharing the experience of illness as well as offering a focus for political action. Thus those suffering illnesses perceived to be caused in some group-related way, such as those acquired from toxic working conditions, can share some experiences at the same time as pursuing claims for compensation.

Professional/client role relationship

So far we have concentrated on the individual sufferer but, as all roles are **complementary**, we need to examine the other side to the sick role relationship – that of the health carer. The carer role adopts degrees of informality, the most formal of these being the clinical role a doctor takes with a patient.

As there are certain obligations and expectations on the role of the patient, so there are special expectations for the role of the professional. The medical practitioner role, as one of the older professional roles, sets a standard by which all other professional roles are judged.

Medical practice has been highly institutionalised in advanced societies. In other words, it is clearly defined in legal, ethical and political terms. A key characteristic of professionalism is an ideology of caring which puts clients' interests first. The caring ethos is designed to help solve clients' problems – to care *about* and *for* – to secure successful outcomes. Professional specialist knowledge should be supported by a body of theory, facts and research. The procedures adopted by the professional are expected to be as objective as possible and not confused with other social relations.

The principle of **detachment** establishes the incorruptibility of the professional. Their relationship to patients is private and confidential. It should be segregated from other public or personal relationships. All of these assumptions permit legitimate access to patients' bodies and minds by relative strangers. External and/or internal interference with patients' bodies through gaze and touch is allowed only in patients' interests. It should be in no-one else's interests, including those of the medical practitioner.

However, in all professional/client meetings there is no simple relationship between expectations, obligations and outcome. Instead, outcomes depend on **definitions of the situation**, which can be redefined during the social interaction. Past events and experiences as much as present circumstances affect both parties' perspectives on the situation and their role performances.

Two sets of situation-defining processes determine outcomes in the professional/client relationship:

1. *Identifying the service to be given* – Both clients and professionals need some idea of what task is to be accomplished. These two perspectives could, of course, be divergent, and much of the initial interaction between the two may be about matching these perspectives.

2. *Identifying the roles to be played by each party* – There is a need to decide not only what the meeting is about, but also how to go about achieving that task. This will call for congruence in role playing and negotiations about role expectations, particularly if there are varying definitions of the situation or conflicting role expectations.

Key questions

As patient or carer, can you recall any incident when complementarity was missing from the role relationship, that is, when the expectations of professional and client did not match, or when definitions of the situation varied?

Power and the patient

Understanding the processes involved in entering and playing the sick role shows that power does not lie with the health professional alone. As we suggested in Chapter 2, everyone has or can gain access to some political resources. Both the patient and significant others who are in a position to react to the patient's reports about their feelings can apply power in the professional/client relationship. The physician's clinical response to feelings of illness is to use their power(s) to identify physical causes for the complaint, legitimise the sick status of the individual and then seek and apply treatment. It is the interaction between all participants in the role play that determines outcomes.

However, the health care encounter also has to be understood within a broader social framework. Institutionalised health care is a form of **social control** through legitimising or challenging clients' feelings. Awareness of the generalised other and the larger expectations of society intervenes in the supposed private relationship between professional and clients. It is not that the patient has no power, but there remains an **uneven distribution of power** between professional and client in the clinical relationship, particularly when the patient is unconscious.

Some clients see health care professionals as 'agents' of the authorities or representative of officialdom. This may be due to clients' previous dissatisfaction with outcomes, confrontational experiences with other professionals or even a general view about the relationship between health and care workers and the state. If professionals assume responsibility for maintaining public health, those who threaten the welfare of the community by their attitudes and practices are seen to be in need of control.

This is a dilemma which social workers have recognised for some time and why social work approaches cover the political spectrum. These range from the authoritarian who keeps an eye on clients' behaviour with a view to controlling it, to the radical worker who sees many clients' problems arising out of inadequacies of public provision and attempts actively to involve themselves in community problems.

Given the expectation that professionals will provide impartial advice and offer impersonal treatment, clients may be disturbed by an overinformal attitude on the part of the professional. Family physicians who make jokes may unsettle a patient who is expecting something entirely different. It is for this type of reason that gynaecological examinations are ceremonialised or ritualised.

Professionals' expectations about clients can alter if clients show themselves to be more knowledgeable than was originally thought. This amounts to a change in the perceived status of the client and happens when health care professionals themselves seek medical care.

In routine work settings, professionals often adopt mechanisms to mark membership boundaries. In formal health care settings the protection of the boundaries to membership is maintained by receptionists. Certain markers are taken as proof of membership: speaking with a particular accent or vocabulary, clothing (perhaps uniforms) or carrying articles of equipment. Conversely, there are some disadvantaging markers which are taken as signifying 'non-membership', such as being accompanied by young children. This makes it difficult to act authoritatively or to be identified as having an authoritative role in many official settings. This offers an important clue to some of the disadvantages suffered by informal carers when they attempt to play a visible, active part in health care settings.

Patients wearing either ordinary clothes or bedtime wear, or lacking a medical vocabulary, may feel very much outsiders. Conversely, health or medical trainees or long-term patients gain skills and knowledge which enable them to participate confidently within medical settings. The comfortable familiarity with such markers displayed by professionals can be the very thing which makes the outsider – the client – feel uncomfortable.

Conclusion

Co-operation is a reciprocal process. Your rights depend on others fulfilling their obligations to you and vice versa. This reciprocal process of complementarity is fundamental to role relationships. Thus the playing of the role of 'father' depends on the playing of the role of 'son'. The role of 'nurse' depends on the role of 'patient'. Each role position entails both rights and duties.

The concept of role is a common-sense analytical tool which is used in an everyday manner by ordinary members of society in order to regulate their mutual expectations of one another. A role concept enables us to anticipate or predict the ways in which people are likely to behave, so that we can adjust our own behaviour accordingly.

To see our behaviour contained in roles need not deprive us of our individuality. We are all unique, but we all have to engage in socially patterned activities. Personality, which makes us different, is composed of socialisation and social interaction. The socialised self is reinforced or altered in each new interaction. Our uniqueness is something we construct with the assistance of others. The most significant others in our early lives are to be found in our family and household. The most fundamental understanding we have of power and control in caring relationships can be found in the experiences we gain in acquiring basic family roles; it is this set of experiences we consider next.

Further reading

Duck, S. (1991) *Human Relationships*, 2nd edn, London: Sage.
A readable and clear book on communication and roles.

Furnham, A. and Stacey, B. (1991) *Young People's Understanding of Society*, London: Routledge.
An attempt at 'reciprocating our cognition' about youth.

Silverman, D. (1987) *Communication and Medical Practice* (Social Relations in the Clinic) London: Sage.
Raises role relationship issues in the context of communication practices.

Chapter 4 The Basis of Informal Care: Families and Households

People do things in, for and because of families. Families are like miniature societies in controlling and distributing resources, particularly those connected with health and caring. However, we cannot assume that we know what a family is and what families do. Even though families are found in most societies throughout the world they are not organised in the same way. It is difficult to describe a typical family setting. Parenting styles and household amenities differ according to variations in family types, class, ethnic background and local circumstances. Comparisons between societies in terms of how they organise their family life show us a great deal about how the rest of that society works.

Family nature and functions

> A **family** is a group of persons directly linked by kin connections, the adult members of which assume responsibility for caring for children. **Kinship ties** are connections between individuals, established either through marriage, or through the lines of descent that connect blood relatives... **Marriage** can be defined as a socially-acknowledged and approved sexual union between two adult individuals.
>
> (Giddens 1997: 140)

Caring responsibilities are often organised by members of **households,** and the kind of family we regard as typical is only one of these.

Households are groups of individuals who live at the same address and share their living accommodation... a family is a household in which a man and woman live alone or together with their dependent child(ren) sharing a common system of housekeeping.

(Graham 1984: 19)

Whatever the precise definition, these are **groupings of individuals based on biological descent, economic co-operation and/or common residence.**
Functionalist theorists explain the universal existence of such groups by looking at the basic biological and physiological needs of humans which may have produced families. The need for:

- reproduction – expressed in sex drives in the individual;
- nutrition – to find or produce food in order to eat;
- protection from the environment – the natural environment and other humans;
- care of the absolutely dependent human infant.

You may say that these basic needs are what led humans into creating societies, and that is really what a family is – the most fundamental form of human society.

Key questions

As a way of reflecting on how important families are to society, think about what a society without family groups would look like. Aldous Huxley's *Brave New World* offers one fictional example.

To create a family-free society we would have to construct a system in which our biological parents were never known to us. Babies would have to be conceived and developed outside the womb or children separated from their biological parents at birth. Primary socialisation would still have to be provided so that people knew how to behave in their society, and children would have to be economically supported until they could fend for themselves. This says nothing about the need to provide the means of sexual gratification, unless the sex drive were suppressed.

The Soviet Union attempted to get rid of the family as a unit after the Russian Revolution of 1917. Attempts have been made to establish communes, often in order to avoid some aspects of family life. Israeli Kibbutzim have applied some of these principles, but socially regulated patterns of mating still exist there and children are recognised as the offspring of particular couples.

The family does more than meet the individual physiological needs mentioned above. It also attends to the social and cultural needs of societies. A range of social functions which are fulfilled by the family are:

- **Economic** – controlling wealth and income, seeking work and the consumption of goods;

- **Political** – providing political socialisation, establishing patterns of authority and maintaining principles of inheritance;

- **Communal** – integrating tribal or kinship identity and forming local networks of relationship for caring, for allocation of resources and for friendship;

- **Cultural** – passing on values and standards, setting norms of acceptable behaviour and establishing leisure activities;

- **Sexual** – controlling sexual relationships and human reproduction.

Together these functions show how families are **sites of learning and caring**.

Key questions

How else could these functions be fulfilled?

As a result of the growth of complex industrial society families now have limited functions and hold a less vital position in society. Individual achievement through other institutions which exist in education, leisure and the workplace are more important in fulfilling these functions.

Many of us still retain mythic imagery about the value of family life in spite of doubts about its contemporary relevance and despite evidence of its problematic nature. Politicians of varying persuasions have promoted the value of family life by constructing images of a utopia based upon historic fictions about the harmonious family in history.

On the other hand, writers, poets, psychiatrists and others have expressed serious reservations about the damage caused by families:

> Far from being the basis of the good society, the family, with its narrow privacy and tawdry secrets, is the source of all our discontents.
>
> (Leach 1967)

In the 1960s, the anti-psychiatrist R.D. Laing and his colleague Aaron Esterson (Laing and Esterson 1970) suggested that certain forms of schizophrenia originated in family oppression, while David Cooper (1972) actively promoted the demise of the family.

Exercise

Find out, by asking people, what sorts of image of the family they hold.

How is that imagery constructed?

What meanings do such images have for individuals who are members of a family or household and for those who are not?

To do this exercise you will need to find out: what 'models' do we have of family life; do different sorts of people have different 'model families' in mind; and do we compare ourselves with some families and not others?

Family forms in history

Young and Willmott (1961, 1975) conducted over twenty years of research into the nature of family life in the UK. They offer a four-stage overview of the development of the family for the past two hundred years. In the first stage – the **pre-industrial family** – the husband and wife and unmarried children worked together as a domestic unit of agricultural and textile production. Work was home based and labour intensive.

This was gradually supplanted as a consequence of the industrial and agricultural revolutions of the eighteenth century by the **early industrial family**. With the growth of the factory system the family stopped being a production unit and became wage dependent. Wages were low, employment uncertain and poverty rife. So family networks **extended** as a safeguard against economic insecurity. The extension was focused upon females, mainly mothers and daughters, and became a tight-knit network which largely excluded the males. Thus the men took to the local inn for the conviviality and social solidarity that was missing from home. Role segregation between men and women in the domestic context naturally followed, and this extended to life outside the home.

However, the family historian Peter Laslett (1977) has spent much of his career questioning ideas about what life was like before and during industrialisation. He has countered notions of an idyllic, rural life in which everything was provided for, the sun always shone and the crops always grew. His research suggests that from 1564 to 1821 only about 10 per cent of households contained kin beyond the basic nuclear family comprising parents and their immediate children. He showed that the **nuclear family** has been the typical family unit throughout Western Europe for many centuries, contrasting markedly with domestic structures in Eastern Europe and Asia.

Young and Wilmott (1975) claimed the emergence of the **symmetrical family** as the third stage of family development. As families moved away from close working-class communities and became more geographically mobile and more affluent (from the late 1950s through to the 1960s), their old network ties were broken and families became more home based. Affluence came from better job security, higher real wages, women taking paid work and the provision of improved welfare benefits. This all reduced economic insecurity. With cars, foreign holidays and home-based leisure, there was less unevenness in conjugal roles. Family size reduced to the nuclear family, and people became more instrumental and materialistic in their values.

This view was challenged by Elizabeth Bott's (1971) study of **conjugal role relations** – the division of labour between marital partners – revealing differences between middle- and working-class practices. While middle-class roles became more equal, this was not the case with working-class partnerships. Whether or not spouses shared domestic tasks depended on the degree of connection of their other social networks. The working classes tended to retain extended family networks and related attitudes and domestic practices. Ann Oakley (1984) similarly found class differentials in conjugal roles, although few men had a high level of participation in housework and childcare. Few marriages were truly egalitarian.

There is an implication in Young and Willmott's work that the middle and upper classes take the lead in setting family patterns and that the lower classes follow as their circumstances change. For example, divorce used to be only something the upper and middle classes could do or even afford; as the laws changed and the costs reduced so the working classes started doing it too. Thus the fourth stage of family development entails **stratified diffusion**, in which upper-class family practices get gradually diffused down the class hierarchy. Thus Young and Wilmott believed that the increasingly work-centred lives that the middle classes engage in spread to working-class family structures. This introduces more symmetry in tasks performed by husband and wife, and less reliance on extended family support. The problem with this is that the working classes are less likely to be able to afford the costs of substituting the care and support resources which were once supplied by the extended family (Arber and Ginn 1992).

Inequalities and difference

Studies of poverty, ill health or homelessness have linked social disadvantages with home circumstances, and mothers are frequently blamed for their failure to perform particular roles adequately. This assumes that the role of the female parent in learning and caring is crucial.

Feminist critiques of such blame-placing have stressed that many concepts of family function are based on stereotypes that are not universal. Feminists question the assumption that families are necessarily benevolent and harmonious units, and that mothers are necessarily expert carers. Marriage and family life often put particular strains on women because roles within marriage are not only different, but also unequal. The organisation of family life reflects the distribution of power between men and women. The allocation of unpaid caring roles to women fits neatly with ideas of women as a reserve army of labour who may be removed from employment when the labour market no longer requires extra hands. Yet in lower-class households where male partners' incomes are not able to support all members, women's dependence through lack of an independent income is greatly increased.

Social differences cut across patterns of family experiences. What parents see as appropriate goals and methods in socialisation are highly dependent on their culture. For example, deference to authority has traditionally been highly valued by members of the lower classes. Their parenting styles have been observed to be more controlling and authoritarian, with less dialogue between parents and children about the reasons for rules. In contrast, middle- and upper-class parenting styles are more democratic and permissive, more likely to support the development of children's creativity, curiosity and self-control. Social class differences in childrearing practices may well reflect parents' own social experiences. At work, working-class adults are often required to follow instructions set by supervisors who seldom explain the reasons for rules.

Marxist perspectives on the family have emphasised how the family structure contributes to reproducing the relations of capitalism. Within the family hierarchy, experiences of childhood submission to parents establish the basis for obedience in adults. The ideology of breadwinning and the inescapability of working for a living provides the necessary motivation to work.

Inequalities in the relative power of different family members may be reinforced through physical violence, although control tends to be much more subtle. Issues around the relative power of different family members even arise in middle-class families, as the writings of some Victorian women have suggested:

> The family uses people, not for what they are, nor for what they are intended to be, but for what it wants them for – its own uses.... If it wants someone to sit in the drawing room, that someone is supplied by the family, though that member may be destined for science or for education or for active superintendance by God, that is, by the gifts within. This system dooms some minds to incurable infancy, others to silent misery. (Nightingale 1860)

Diversity in families and households

Modern family life in most Western industrial societies is now organised in many different ways. The **nuclear family** comprising parents and their children living in one household is now the arrangement for only 40 per cent of people in the UK. In most traditional societies the nuclear family is embedded within much larger kinship networks. **Extended** families are those in which other family members besides the married couple and children live in the same household or in close and continuous contact. **Modified extended families** are those which live apart geographically but maintain regular contact and support through visiting and modern communications. **Single-parent families** are now increasingly common. In 1990 20 per cent of all families with dependent children in the UK were single-parent families, largely as a result of divorce. However, in 30 per cent of single-parent families headed by women the mothers had not married the biological father of their children, and this category of family is increasing. The **reconstituted family** is one in which one or both partners have been previously married and bring with them children from a previous marriage. This reconstructs the family into a **bi-nuclear family** with step-parents and step-children involved in joint custody and co-parenting. In 1990 10 per cent of children lived in step-families following their parents' remarriage. Other kinds of reconstituted family may involve other kin such as grandparents or older brothers or sisters taking on parental roles.

Other household trends show increasing numbers of people living alone, one-parent families and childless married couples. Although the divorce rate has increased, **serial monogamy** remains the current trend. If people seek new partners, they only do so one at a time. This suggests values which no longer emphasise a necessary permanence in intimate relationships. Nonetheless, instability in marital relationships may lead to emotional disturbances, foster a sense of guilt or responsibility in children for any marital breakdown and increase the stress and emotional insecurity of all family members, particularly for single parents with dependent children. All this contributes towards broader changes in gender roles.

Exercise

Consider the family or household structures which you have experienced. How do they compare to the structures discussed above? How is power distributed in the households of which you have experience?

To conduct this analysis look at the distribution of political resources discussed in Chapter 2. Look at how resources are distributed between men and women, between young and old and so on. Consider also the various social roles played by different members of the family or household and how they relate to each other as discussed in Chapter 3.

The focal position of the family as a social institution is seen by the way in which it affects and is affected by broader social trends. A higher divorce rate may reduce the stigma of divorce. Similarly, there is less stigma on pregnancies outside marriage. Durable marriage is not assumed to be inevitable, women are giving birth later in life and single-person households are becoming more common. Same-sex intimate relationships and non-kin multi-adult households further complicate the picture. One could ask whether these are still, recognisably, families or whether families are simply defined by the tasks they undertake, creating household communities of care and support.

Caring still goes on in new household organisations. Indeed, some of them may have been established by the participants to escape the oppression of kinship. Moral communities of attachment may develop around the household or may be focused on systems of mutual support outside domestic arrangements. Intimate relationships can then grow based on these new attachments. One example of this derives from the support arrangements for HIV and AIDS sufferers. The experience of stigma, pain and death has given rise to a sophisticated culture of survival, particularly among gay men, in which **buddying** (the informal but carefully structured system of individual support for the sick or dying) has become symbolic of new forms of solidarity. It may be that buddies fulfil a caring function which would once have been expected from the family.

Key questions

Make a list of the different ways in which people may experience family life in future. What other ways may caring be informally learned and supported in the future?

Ideals and reality

Members of these new types of household may feel deprived of the idealised lifestyle of the mythical family frequently constructed by the media. As they fail to live up to this unattainable image they may feel frustrated or stigmatised. Those people who do not live in families may feel inadequate and that they are missing something.

The artificial image of family life is widely exploited to draw people in to health fads or fashions. Diet and lifestyle habits and attitudes are frequently cultivated for commercial purposes in relation to this idealised image. This may seem acceptable if done for sound health promotional reasons, although it could become a device to market health-related consumer goods. The danger is that such advertising tactics may exclude those who do not fit this conventional imagery.

Reconstituted families may feel that there is something wrong with them when they confront the normal problems of holding a family together, of maintaining links with natural parents and of financial strain. Such experiences may discourage people from wanting to join or make families.

Health professionals need to remain aware of the gap between expectations or idealised imagery and the realities of family and household living. They should certainly not accept at face value stereotypical images about how families lead their lives but should recognise that certain health and care problems may arise out of many kinds of household living arrangement.

It is clear that marriage and family life are not unproblematic institutions. Equality in marriage may be talked about and anticipated but not necessarily realised. Surveys consistently report the view that mothers take more responsibility for children's health, food and clothing than do fathers. Women still spend more time than men on household management work such as washing and ironing, cooking and cleaning. There are pointers that some inequalities within marriage are being tackled, but rising juvenile delinquency and divorce rates are still seen as indicators of some of the failures of marriage-based families as social institutions. Few welfare and social security arrangements take adequate account of radical new family structures.

Exercise

Look at some television soap operas – how is family and household life represented?

Collect health educational and promotional literature, as well as literature selling health goods and services, and look at the family or household imagery employed.

In both cases, are families represented as typical in any way? How is variety in household arrangements represented?

Perhaps one of the best illustrations in recent years of the gap between ideals and reality was the debate in the UK about child sexual abuse following the revelations and enquiries in Cleveland. Here we have the meeting point of many of the actors and themes in debates and constructions about marriage and the family in the 1980s. These include social workers, medical practitioners, the police, the Church, politicians, journalists and the media. The themes include relationships between adults and children and between men and women, the boundaries between the public and the private as they apply to the family, feminism, and professional interventions. The Cleveland case highlights divisions and contradictions in understandings of the family which do not fit ideas about symmetrical families or companionate marriages.

Families and care

The trends we have been discussing suggest considerable alterations of traditional family roles and statuses and the networks of care expected from families. Extended families cannot be relied on for child care: both parents may be breadwinners and children may hold increased status within the family. If women are working, their work is likely to be lower paid. Unemployed men confront role and status changes within the household, and male dominance may be challenged.

Economic resources are often low for many new family types. The physical and psychological health of children may be lowered if both parents are employed outside the domestic environment, while unemployment may lead to conflict and stress within the household. Extended families may live at great geographical distances and cannot be assumed to be available for home care and/or visiting. Formal home help may be needed. Some parents may not be present within the household. Step-and/or biological parents may need to be told separately about children's illnesses. Effective work within primary health care teams requires recognition of these issues. Ironically, the role of family as main carer of the sick has dwindled while governments aim to rebuild this role through community care policies. Alternative networks of support will become essential because of such changes in family structures.

Conclusion: Families, households and health

As a primary socialisation agency the family performs a vital cultural role in the attitudes it engenders towards health. Thus it can promote or discourage health in the field of diet and nutrition, recreation or leisure and the take-up of health care facilities such as immunisation programmes, regular visits to dentists and opticians, and so on. Health habits and attitudes are initially established and maintained within the domestic environment.

Adults and older children usually take on caring roles. Caring responsibilities include a knowledge of primary care and the recognition of when and how to call for outside assistance. Most informal primary care remains in the hands of female family members. Mothers will be the first to take time off work to adopt this role, depending on whether or not they are the main or sole breadwinner. Single parentage and the decline of extended family links may further increase difficulties in the family's maintenance of primary care responsibilities. If extended care is needed, this could seriously threaten the financial security of the family.

Despite such limitations, families within communities can be of influence. Families can show, by their actions, how to behave and what attitudes to hold within a community. Attendance at clinics, school events, clubs and voluntary associations may be focused around family life. This can work in two ways, and more negative behaviour may also be shared between families. Health professionals must maintain awareness of the effects of family lifestyle and the health-promoting, and demoting, potential of the family.

Key questions

What good health practices did you learn from your own family or household? What bad health habits did you pick up?

Remember that we can also learn good practices by observing the bad habits of others.

Families and households are not the only places where relationships of power and control are established and maintained. This also happens in school. Chapter 5 looks at how the more formalised socialisation experience which goes on in educational institutions may reinforce or alter roles and relationships acquired in primary socialisation.

Further reading

Clark, D. (ed.) (1991) *Marriage, Domestic Life and Social Change: Writings for Jacqueline Burgoyne (1944–88)*, London: Routledge.
Gittins, D. (1985) *The Family in Question*, London: Macmillan.
Jackson, S. (1993) *Family Lives – a Feminist Sociology*, Oxford: Blackwell.
Morgan, D. (1985) *The Family, Politics and Social Theory*, London: Routledge & Kegan Paul.
Perelberg, R.J. and Miller, A.C. (eds) (1990) *Gender and Power in Families*, London: Routledge.

All the above works bring the debate about gender, power and household roles up to date.

Chapter 5 Healthy Learning

Modern developments in health promotion have shown how important it is to understand how people learn about health. We can learn about health in medical consultations. Schools and voluntary organisations run health education sessions. Learning goes on in patient self-help groups, in specialist clinics and in antenatal classes.

We often learn more effectively in other, less formal settings. As we discussed in the previous chapter, most learning about health takes place almost incidentally in the networks of care which operate in families and households, and in communities or neighbourhoods. Both as patients and as health care professionals we are learning all the time, and sometimes we learn the wrong things. Bad practice is something we are not always aware of until someone tells us otherwise or something goes wrong. It is for this reason that there have been campaigns to create awareness of good health practices in everyday life. The idea of creating the 'healthy school' or the 'healthy hospital' acknowledges the effects of more subtle learning processes and draws attention to the need to control hidden learning experiences in various ways. First we need to look at how and why learning is formally organised in most societies.

What is schooling for?

Schools are organisations whose purpose is education. In modern societies schooling is the next major socialising influence on children's lives after their family. It is a formally organised learning experience which is compulsory by law between certain ages. Formal education can begin earlier in kindergarten or nursery schools, and for some it never ends.

Schools are frequently the first large organisations with which children have contact. They provide early experiences of formal social settings and of hierarchies of power. Thus, in addition to formal lessons, children also learn about how to behave towards people who have power or status. School provides a **secondary socialisation** process which supplements, but may also challenge, the primary socialisation begun by the family.

Exercise

Make two lists:

● reasons why you went to school;

● reasons why you are in the education system now.

Education serves the purposes of both individuals and society. Individual reasons for wanting education may include fulfilling ambitions for improved job opportunities, personal reward or responding to state or family obligations. On a societal level education prepares people to match the needs of the labour market, to participate in social life or to keep young people usefully occupied when out of the job market. It may even be seen as a large child care agency, caring for children while parents get on with their work.

Analysing education systems

Education systems can be analysed by asking questions about the principal tasks which they face:

1. **Administration** – how is the system managed?

2. **Finance** – where does the money come from?

3. **Access or selection** – how is education to be allocated? How does the system choose who is to be educated and to what level?

4. **Curriculum** – what counts as appropriate knowledge? What is seen as worth knowing and how is that knowledge organised?

5. **Pedagogy** – how is knowledge transmitted or taught?

6. **Assessment** – how are learners tested for their ability?

7 **Evaluation or audit** – how effective is the system in achieving its goals?

In reality, these questions overlap. For example, how we are taught and tested will influence our view of what we are learning, so that pedagogy, assessment and evaluation have critical influences on the curriculum. Similarly, politicians are not content merely to debate the relative importance of arts and literature in the curriculum as against science and technology. They seek to control it on the grounds that they see different forms of knowledge as vital for a society's economic, cultural and political development.

Indeed, when we ask 'Who controls education?', 'Why do they control it?' and 'Who should control it?', we are considering what difference it would make if educational authorities were democratically elected or if they were appointed by central government. Deciding what forms of knowledge are important might be a crucial control issue. So should non-elected professional educators be in control since they are assumed to know what they are talking about? What role is there for the clients in controlling the educational system? Who, in fact, are the clients? Are they the students or parents, or the government, or employers for whom the knowledge and skills are destined?

There has always been tension between centralised and localised control of education, local and national issues, and specialist and general concerns. Locally, people may want schools which maintain their own culture and produce knowledgeable and skilled people who can contribute to and develop the local economy. Central government claims to have a broader overview of national and international economic trends so is better placed to determine future requirements for the whole society. This debate is often coloured by who is paying for the service; does most of the money come from central or from local taxation?

Exercise

Apply these analytic criteria to your own educational experiences.

For each educational setting you were in look at its organisation and how it was financed. How did you gain access to it? Was there competition for places? Were you selected or did you freely choose the organisation? What curriculum was on offer? How were you taught? How were you assessed? Did you participate in evaluations of the learning experience?

Compare this with the educational experiences of your friends, family or colleagues.

There may be significant differences between people according to how each of these analytic questions are dealt with. Experiences vary according to the rural or urban setting of the educational organisation, the size of the organisation, religious affiliations, geographic regions or who pays.

Functions of formal education

Governments and educationalists see formal education as crucial to a society's development. A full understanding of how education works is essential to the successful implementation of social policies and the maintenance of established cultural traditions. Sociologists often express this importance in terms of the fundamental **functions** or purposes of formal education. These functions can be:

- **cultural** – the passing on of accepted values, together with the general knowledge and attitudes appropriate to the correct forms of behaviour in that society;

- **economic** – the teaching of particular skills and knowledge by which individuals can earn themselves a living and contribute to the material welfare of their society;

- **political** – the cultivation of an ordered society in which individuals learn their place in society's decision-making processes;
- **moral** – by which individuals are taught society's basic codes for distinguishing between right and wrong.

Societies may give different emphasis to each of these functions. At some stages in their historical development societies may be less concerned with culture and more interested in the political education of their citizens. Educational institutions may vary in their performance of these fundamental functions between cultivating economic skills or moral development.

Rarely are these functions performed separately. For example, one of the economic functions of education is to prepare people for work. It is commonly assumed that a labour force needs to be provided with some generic skills such as literacy and numeracy. Other skills are more specific to occupations, but a labour force also has to be socialised into work disciplines and the requirements of work organisations, which is essentially a political function.

Exercise

Look at each of the educational institutions you attended and decide which of these functions were being addressed, how they were performed and in what combination.

Consider how these functions relate to education about health.

Is health education a moral, economic, political or cultural matter?

Growth of compulsory mass education

Contemporary educational philosophies, ideologies and practices have their roots in the political, economic and social events of history. Large-scale educational expansion began in the nineteenth century. The population explosion and the growth of urbanisation made clear the deficiencies of educational provision. Owing to the influence of *laissez-faire* doctrines on politics and society, governments were initially reluctant to interfere in educational affairs. Pressure for government intervention in educational provision grew with the recognition by the state and industrialists that continued economic growth – the health of the nation – depended on the development of an adequate system of technical education.

The USA and Germany provided global models for this. Their success in the face of the UK's relative economic decline was due to their advanced systems of technical education. Pressure for UK public education came from the new middle classes, which had emerged with the growth of trade and industry, and were concerned for the occupational and social advancement of their children. Equally important was the threat to government of a radical working class made politically effective by their own forms of education. In the UK, for example, reports from the Schools Inspectorate suggested that, unless a national system of education was provided, the working classes would succumb to more disruptive forms of education with revolutionary implications. Thus a middle-class system of education was established which provided bourgeois facts and values to counteract the dissemination of revolutionary ideas begun by working-class activist groups (Corrigan 1979).

This system had the effect of persuading people to come to terms with a class-based society, to learn to know one's place and the reason for it. Working-class culture – its habits, traditions, ways of speaking and taking leisure – was criticised and replaced by a middle-class morality. In addition, the growing factory system required punctuality and a much tighter discipline from its workforce. A school system based on an hierarchical ideology and rigid discipline suited the production of an obedient labour force.

The system of compulsory mass education we accept so readily in advanced industrial societies was a deliberate attempt to control the masses and keep industry fuelled for economic and political purposes. This happened in both capitalist and communist societies for similar reasons. Formal education systems do not emerge from the ideas put forward by educationists. Instead there are several groups of stakeholders, each seeking their own cultural, economic, moral and political goals. Taken together, this amounts to their own educational ideology, a particular view about what education is for and what can be achieved by formalising it.

For these reasons there have been many attempts to impose uniformity on education systems. Whether variety or consistency should be sought in education is a subject for debate. On the one hand, uniformity is needed so that the system can be understood and adequately used by all members of society. Parents advise their children, students select an appropriate career path and employers make comparisons between the abilities of job candidates based on their qualifications. Similarly, any attempts to apply principles of **equality of educational opportunity** requires that whoever you are and wherever you live, you can be sure of acquiring as good an educational provision as the next person. On the other hand, variety may permit more freedom of choice. Educational provision can be selected according to individual needs rather than forcing students into an unsuitable category. Equality needs to be balanced against **parity of esteem**, by which different educational organisations are seen as fulfilling different functions and none is necessarily seen as superior to another.

Governments have, in recent years, subjected their educational systems to harsh economies. In spite of that they still hold the view that education and economic growth are linked and arrange post-compulsory education training schemes with this in mind. Demographic peaks and troughs continue to affect educational requirements and provision. Educational institutions are encouraged to be more flexible in terms of numbers of permanent staff employed, class sizes and teacher:pupil ratios.

Key questions

This debate about who controls and why is vital when applied to the education of health care professionals. So too is the dilemma of uniformity versus diversity. Thus learning theory suggests that autonomous learners are more effective, but this means that learners will learn different things at different paces and at different times. Can this really be allowed for health care professionals whose licence to practise essentially claims that they are

cont'd

---

competent to perform certain tasks? Medical education is moving towards problem-centred learning and away from the more formal didactic forms of learning. The ultimate test often lies in the assessment system, the great leveller.

What do you think? How important is it that all health care professionals are taught the same curriculum in the same way? If not all the curriculum is held in common, which elements are essential?

Inequality in education

Mass education is expensive, and limits have to be put on how many people can be educated to the highest level. As we discuss in detail in Chapter 7, social inequalities arise out of the fact that **valued resources are limited**. Resources have to be distributed among those who want or need them, and some means of allocation has to be devised. This is as true for resources for education and training as it is for health resources.

Educational opportunities, like political resources, are distributed unevenly. We are not all allowed the same amount of time in the formal education system. At each successive stage in the education system, progressively smaller numbers of people survive to enter the next stage. All mass educational systems are **elitist** in this sense, and most countries have had to confront the problem of selection for, or access to, successive educational stages.

Educational inequality exists in terms of differences in individual achievement, in the life chances endowed by varying cultural and economic backgrounds, and in aptitude or ability to learn, which might determine the educational potential of individuals. Learning environments may vary according to local facilities, to school size or with teaching practices. It could be impossible to create a uniform educational experience, no matter how centrally controlled the formal education system.

In some respects inequality in education is an inevitability. Pursuing equality in education would be fruitless. Instead, an **equality of opportunity** is sought. In other words, the debate is about how far it is possible to give everyone the same chances of gaining access to scarce and valued educational resources.

Sociological research has shown that the chances of surviving each successive stage in the educational process vary between different social groups (Rubinstein 1979). Individuals receive different amounts and quality of education according to variables such as class, measured intelligence, gender and ethnicity. What is often missing is an explanation of why this should be so.

Concerns over equality of opportunity and parity of esteem arise most forcibly at entry to secondary education. From initially arguing that education should be offered to all according to need and ability, the former Soviet Union eventually used Communist Party membership of pupils and their parents as a selection criterion, thereby creating an educated elite which controlled the country politically and intellectually. The USA and the UK have attempted to select according to 'objective tests' of intellectual ability. The principle is that tests of children can be used to predict the benefits gained from investing in their long-term education. Such tests have been seen as a process of allocation rather than a competitive examination. In practice, success at such tests gave access to the better schools and therefore better chances of academic success.

Key questions

Access to most health care professional courses are competitive. Do you think this selection process operates a principle of equality of opportunity? Should it? Can the selection procedure be improved?

Theoretical variations

The theoretical traditions of functionalist, interactionist and conflict perspectives offer different sets of explanations for the existence of educational inequalities. They vary in their recommendations or prescriptions for how education ought to be organised. There are surprising overlaps in the practical solutions offered to educational problems by theorists from different traditions.

Functionalist theorists see education as vital in socialising the young into acceptance of society's dominant norms and values. If school examinations encourage individual success through graded qualifications, this fits with a modern society which is fundamentally unequal, individualistic and competitive. Students learn conformity and how to behave in competitively hierarchical institutions.

Since education imparts knowledge which is useful for the economic system, the selection of those appropriate for particular social roles is important. Occupational status is frequently allocated on the basis of educational achievement, so the education system selects and qualifies according to demonstrated ability. Functionalists argue that a society's survival depends on its ability to inspire the best people to strive to reach the key positions. The education system has a vital role in allocating and inspiring people to seek to fulfil these tasks.

This view has been criticised for ignoring the existing unequal distribution of socially desirable traits. Status and class groups often preserve rewards for themselves and their descendants rather than for the benefit of society at large. An approach based on merit only works if the class system is open. Not everyone aspires to educational success nor values knowledge and training; only those brought up to do so are likely to achieve such educational success.

For this reason the **interactionist** perspective has focused on the student's reaction to the process of education. Students' background culture – their values, norms, attitudes and beliefs – frame their educational experience. Only in this way will the cultural resistance of some groups to the dominant educational forms of success be understood. From this viewpoint it has been argued that everyone should have equal educational opportunities at the start of the process. Competition will still result in unequal examination results and different career opportunities at later stages. A **compensatory education** of this sort seeks to promote equality of opportunity while allowing the inevitability of educational inequality.

Conflict perspectives underline how inequalities within schools reflect those in the wider society and are critical of approaches which encourage conformity to capitalist forms of organisation. They consider that the functioning of the educational system is largely determined by the needs of the capitalist socio-economic system, which does not match people to occupations either effectively or fairly. Education in such a society contributes to the continuance of class inequalities. Socialisation in this context means that the majority of working-class children who fail academically tend to accept their own failure and the success of the middle-class children as legitimate. The success of a minority of working-class children fosters the illusion of a neutral or fair educational system.

Socially structured inequality in education

Educational success has been shown to be linked to social factors such as class, gender and ethnicity. The material and cultural disadvantages which limit the possibilities for educational achievement are based on household resources, family lifestyles. and the abilities and interest of parents.

Bernstein (1975) studied how language use in different cultural groups might affect their educational potential. He argues that groups vary in their **family role control systems**, that is, in their ways of controlling family roles. Different family role control systems produce different language uses or 'codes'. **Restricted** codes have everyday informal speech patterns and produce a **collective** orientation toward the community. **Elaborated** codes use more abstract, conceptual language and are more **individualistic** in orientation. Middle-class children are more likely to encounter elaborated codes in speech used at home and thus gain competency in the sorts of vocabulary and language employed in the school environment. This continuity between the cultures of school and home gives them an advantage over working-class children, whose home experiences contrast sharply with those of school. Bernstein suggests that working-class pupils have to leave their identity at the school gate.

This view was challenged by Labov (1969), who found that black working-class children were capable of expressing themselves in abstract conceptual terms once they felt comfortable and confident. However, the contradictions between school and home cultures remain. This partly explains variations in the levels of attainment of children from different ethnic groups in multicultural societies. The relatively high success rates of children from Asian families, compared with Afro-Caribbeans, in the UK is also explained by social class differences. Most Asian immigrants were middle class in culture and in aspirations, whereas most Afro-Caribbean male immigrants went into manual occupations. Asian communities have typically placed a high value on educational achievement and give active family support to children's studies.

Variations in educational achievement are also linked to gender differences. Abbott and Wallace (1990) report how, since the 1940s, girls have consistently outperformed boys in the early years of formal education, but the gap narrows so that males are more likely to do well at college or university and after. Indeed, females and males perform differently in different subjects. Female students perform most strongly in professions allied to medicine, arts, languages and biology, while a higher proportion of male students succeed in computer science, engineering, technology, mathematics, physics and chemistry.

Key questions

Think about your own educational achievement, and that of your colleagues and friends:

What are the markers of a successful educational career?

How do educational achievements affect subsequent life and health chances?

What educational inequalities of gender, class, ethnicity or age have you seen and/or experienced?

Consider how your background has influenced your educational experiences. What discouraged and encouraged you within formal education? Consider the educational values which were espoused within your community. How much more do you know about your life and health as a result of your educational experiences?

Formal educational knowledge is not neutral but reflects traditional masculine assumptions about expertise, competition and individualism. For example, medical schools are dominated by male values and culture. Females who succeed have to assimilate a masculine culture, and this accounts for the relatively higher drop-out rate of female medical students. Nurse education reverses this bias, and it may be just as hard for male students to survive the traditional ethos of a nursing curriculum.

Genetic endowment – the IQ debate

A recurrent debate has been whether some individuals possess innate qualities (by **'nature'**) which give them better chances of educational success, or whether social environment (**'nurture'**) can improve upon nature.

One side of the argument is that some people are more intelligent than others and that intelligence is measurable using an **intelligence quotient** (IQ). If intelligence is largely innate, there is little that can be done to improve it. It should be accurately measurable at an early age, and educational resources can be applied to those with ability rather than wasted on those without it. The alternative view is that we can improve on those innate abilities by acquiring more opportunity and potential from our social environment. Not only would it be iniquitous to remove privilege from some people on the basis of early IQ measures, but it is also wasteful not to allow other creative human qualities to emerge and be developed by the education system.

It is difficult to measure intelligence separately from other qualities such as attention span, motivation, relevance or anxiety, which may vary across cultures, between individuals and even according to the mood or particular situation of an individual at any one time. Rose and Rose (1979) show how, while IQ scores correlate highly with educational success, they are environmentally influenced and predict formal academic achievement rather than future intellectual competence. IQ tests are culturally biased in not measuring the things that are valued in different environments. They do not measure the spatial judgement abilities of the Inuit people, the intuitive navigational skills of South Sea islanders nor the ability of the Kikuyu to count large cattle herds at a glance. More subtle subcultural variations within industrial societies may have been missed. If so, any concentration of educational resources on some groups rather than others is misguided and unfair.

Attempts to detect intellectual ability at an early age are based on a misunderstanding of the nature of human learning. Humans acquire some abilities genetically, but other abilities emerge out of interaction with the physical and cultural environment, and there is no reliable way of separating out these qualities. Measuring the balance between them serves no useful purpose in terms of educational policy. More recently, researchers have suggested that, instead of measuring intelligence, we should explore multiple intelligences. We have to understand the combination of linguistic, logical, mathematical, musical, spatial, kinesic, mechanical, clerical and reasoning skills that a person possesses, some of which come from nature and others of which may have been nurtured.

Key questions

Have you observed qualities of intellect in yourself or in others which are difficult to quantify?

Are they valued or not within formal educational settings?

Deschooling and radical alternatives to formal education

There is an implicit assumption that compulsory education for the masses is inevitable in a complex industrial society. Yet it is evident that public education is conducted in the interests of those who already possess economic and political power, and existing inequalities continue to be reproduced. A radical critique of state compulsory mass education has come from a **deschooling** movement which questions the fundamental assumptions of formal schooling. Deschooling writers argue for an expansion of informal educational opportunities and the creation of a **learning society** in which learning throughout life is fostered in the interests of individual learners.

Lister (1974) summarises the work of the deschooling writers of the 1960s. Goodman thought that the bureaucratic educational system produced fodder for an industrial machine. He wanted to return to more informal learning by experience supported by tutored apprenticeships. Freire argued that mass education is not meaningful for the majority of the population. School fragments and mystifies the world and the masses remain dependent on the system. The oppressed are seen as the pathogens of the healthy society, and this culminates in their being cared for and dependent upon a welfare system which reduces general social problems to individual cases.

Freire wanted intellectuals to aid the masses in perceiving the social, political and economic contradictions in their society. He thought all curricula should directly confront the problems posed by **real-life situations**. Educators and students should work together towards problem-solving knowledge. This sort of education would not be static but a dynamic form of **permanent education**.

Exercise

Apply this approach to the professional/client relationship. The client presents the 'real-life problem' and the knowledge of both the professional and the client is enhanced as they work together towards a solution. Practise some 'role distancing' (see Chapter 3) to imagine how this works.

Informal learning, problem-solving and an attempt to avoid knowledge hierarchies are essential to the success of this exercise.

Another deschooler, Illich, was concerned with the messages of the **hidden curriculum**. This refers to those things which are not consciously taught but involve values or ways of behaving which are implicitly passed on in school procedure and organisation. The overt or **revealed curriculum** is contained in the specific subjects on the timetable. Many of the messages of the hidden curriculum are embodied in school rituals such as dress codes, speech days, badges, trophies and competitions. The hierarchy of authority within the school, relationships between teachers and students and the physical layout of the classroom all implicitly 'teach' what count as appropriate attitudes, values and behaviour. Such messages inculcate work disciplines such as hard work, keeping time, obeying authority, identification with nationality, moral codes, acceptable work behaviour and dress, roles and stereotypes.

Some of the more subtle messages include the view that schooling and education are the same thing; thus one is only being educated when in school. The 'real world' comes to be seen as having nothing to do with education, while school is seen as unworldly. There is an assumption that learning is a consequence of teaching, and we do not see learning as taking place in non-educational situations. Esteemed knowledge is assumed to be that which is professionally delivered, validated and certificated, and packaged in an official curriculum. More subtly, it is not only what is explicitly included in a curriculum that teaches us what is to be considered valuable knowledge, but also those things which are neglected or even deliberately omitted: the English literary curriculum neglects African, Asian or Eastern European writers; the medical curriculum excludes some forms of alternative or complementary medicine.

Exercise

List the things you remember learning from the hidden curriculum of your previous formal education.

What messages about good health behaviour are learned in such informal ways, and what bad health practices did you pick up?

List the elements of the hidden curriculum in your present educational experience?

Do any of these hidden learning experiences vary according to gender, class or ethnicity? Compare your own experiences with those of colleagues.

Most of us learn about sexual behaviour, smoking and drug use and abuse from the hidden curriculum. The power of informally learning 'unhealthy' practices from peers, as against what is formally taught about health, is worth considering. How easy is it to counter the bad health lessons embodied in hidden curricula?

Some of the deschooling principles have more recently had a greater chance of being realised since the importance of a permanent education has been recognised in the growth of **continuing professional development**. Gradually, continuing education is becoming formally required for most professional occupations.

> **Key questions**
>
> Considering all these educational issues together:
>
> Would health professionals learn more effectively as apprentices?
>
> Should they work in small groups with a mentor to see them through each educational stage?
>
> Should there be a tiered educational structure, with different professionals educated and qualified to different levels?

One proposition has been that all health professionals should be educated on the same curriculum, with increasing specialism as they move on through the curriculum, stopping at the point which suits the individual but able to continue later on. Thus nurses, doctors, physiotherapists and so on could all receive the same education at first, and where they stopped could determine the level of health care work they were allowed to perform. This would not stop them qualifying further at some later stage. Are there some health professions for which lifelong learning should be a condition of professional practice and some for which it need not be?

Learning about health

Health educators have asked whether school can be a health-promoting agency. This question may be answered using the analytical framework introduced earlier and by considering both the hidden and revealed curriculum of schools.

The formal curriculum may cultivate health knowledge and physical fitness. For example, school formalises public health inspections of children, is implicated in sex and health education and encourages fitness through sport and games activity. But how much of that is counteracted by the less formal observations of the unhealthy behaviour of teachers or peers who may smoke, be obese, eat and drink without nutritional care and show disinterest in sport?

Corrigan (1979) suggests that alienation fostered by school cultivates more 'bad health' habits as a reaction. When taken with poor parental or domestic relationships, truanting from the constraints of school encourages activities such as the use of drugs, alcohol and smoking. The more alienated the child becomes, the more risky the behaviour. Corrigan's argument is that this represents a way in which children use the few political resources they have in order to gain some control over their own lives.

The ability of formal education not to be alienating depends on the depth of the relationship between the school and the community. Thus some regions in both Europe and North America instituted **health-promoting school** campaigns in the early 1990s. They employed holistic perspectives on health and relied upon inter-agency collaboration. There are mechanisms for the audit of health criteria within schools and for healthy alliances with other schools. Without radical alternatives to much that is embedded in formal schooling, the success of such schemes remains in doubt.

Conclusion

Education is supposed to help students become more fully developed through acquiring knowledge and an ability to think, question, communicate effectively and solve problems. Many educational institutions espouse such principles in their mission statements, and many curricula aim to cultivate autonomous, critically aware and reflective learners.

Some aspects of formal educational organisation work against principles of independent personal development. The working conditions and resources of educational organisations are less able to deal with students who are highly individualist, imaginative or creatively intelligent. It could be argued that the imposition of a standardised national curriculum and specific vocational skills training for jobs restricts opportunities for such personal development.

Another argument against a 'personal development' goal for formal education is that it has to be used by society as a means of social control. People cannot be allowed to do as they wish or to learn according to their whims. For economic reasons, if nothing else, it is vital to ensure minimum health standards for the population and to ensure that they gain access to the means of supporting themselves and their families. It could be argued that, by occupying the energy of otherwise unemployed groups, education reduces threats to the stability of the state and the wider society.

The last exercise in this chapter focuses on these issues in a practical way.

Exercise

Consider a health education activity you have observed or taken part in:

What was the aim or intended outcome of this activity?

What groups were intended to gain personal health benefit from the session?

How effective was it in achieving its aims?

What social factors influenced how far these aims were achieved?

Describe how it was organised and who participated. Apply the following analytical categories: administration; finance; access; curriculum; pedagogy; assessment; evaluation.

In what ways did this activity provide its own hidden curriculum or depend upon participants' previous learning? What features of the hidden curriculum do you see as helping the group to gain personal health benefits? Which features hindered health gains?

Use the elements of the hidden curriculum derived earlier, and do not forget such topics as respect for authority, social skills, work-related routines and values associated with particular social groups.

Students in most formal educational settings perceive themselves as having few political resources and little ability to control outcomes. That is why hidden curricula are sometimes seen as forms of resistance. Thus health messages from authoritative sources are undermined by 'unhealthy' practices which become part of student culture – such as drinking alcohol to excess. Most of us are optimistic about acquiring more control when we take up paid employment; the next chapter shows how this has always been harder than we might hope.

Further reading

Harrison, J. and Edwards, J. (eds) (1994) *Developing Health Education in the Curriculum*, London: D. Fulton.
Addresses issues involved with embedding health education in the formal curriculum.

Ogier, M.E. (1989) *Working and Learning: The Learning Environment in Clinical Nursing*, London: Scutari Press.
Looks at how one health profession addresses the problem of formal professional education.

Chapter 6 Working for Health

Work has profound effects on us. Occupations are so important to adults that they affect our health. The nature and conditions of work influence how we give and receive health care. Some kinds of work are highly visible and their effects fairly evident. Working on a building site is labour intensive, dirty, outdoor work. Domestic work is less visible, but informal caring work can be labour intensive, dirty, indoor work. The emotional and health consequences of different kinds of work can be even more invisible. Not having full-time paid work can reduce opportunities to exercise control over whether we live and work in environments which are more or less likely to enhance our health chances. Distinctions drawn between more visible and less visible forms of work have consequences for how work is organised, distributed and rewarded, and attitudes toward housework and care work.

Conceptualising work

Work may be defined as **the carrying out of tasks which involve physical or mental effort**. Work is done to produce goods and services which meet human needs.

Employment entails work done on someone else's instructions and for rewards determined by them. The self-employed, houseworkers and the unemployed can all be working even if they are not paid for it. We use the term 'work' in many different ways to cover **obligated time** which includes activities that are more or less visible, more or less paid, have vocational aims or are part of ordinary life, such as family work.

Employment usually involves highly visible work. It takes place in formal workplaces with clearly designated tasks, resources and symbols (such as a uniform or distinctive working clothes). Responsibilities and higher status are attached to employment. It is usually work which is paid at an agreed rate. Lower status, less visible work often provides the support for more visible types of work. Domestic chores, such as housework, and other informal tasks involve unpaid work, are more often performed by women and are seen as necessary to support the employed worker.

Most of us spend most of our lives working for someone else. We do it largely to earn the financial means for subsistence. We work to eat to live and to enable our families to survive. In so doing we help to fuel an economic system upon which the lives of other people are dependent.

Exercise

Look at the types of work you do. List the kinds of 'employed' work and the 'non-employed' work that you have done. What reasons would you give for doing each type of work?

We do not often think about basic reasons for working. There are many socially shaped reasons for working: the expectations of others that we ought to work, its being a part of our culture, a moral pressure on us that work is a good thing to do and the satisfaction to be gained from completing the work tasks themselves. We may work to seek the company of other people.

Early theories about work

Throughout history major upheavals in society have been linked to changes in the organisation of work. Industrialisation, the growth of bureaucratic organisations, the moves away from traditional rural communities, and working for money rather than the exchange of goods and services have all had major effects on the individual and on society. These remain of vital importance to our working experiences today.

Marx (1864) argued that humans need to work to fulfil the creative potential of their species. He felt that the potential rewards of work should be more than just a matter of surviving but that the conditions produced by industrial capitalism had perverted the nature of work and prevented people from gaining fulfilment from it. The capitalist system geared to maximising profits and efficiency produced inhuman working environments: factories, mills and mines in which humans were debased. Marx pointed to degrading conditions of work which created low pay and led to poor living conditions. People had no time or resources left for themselves to freely choose their work and leisure activities. They barely had time or resources to reproduce the labour force in order to fuel the economic system.

In Marx's view the organisation of work was a form of social control, keeping us all occupied, with time or space neither for raising our intellectual abilities nor for political dissent. This control worked in the interests of those groups most able to profit under such a system. Marx and his followers held a view of work organisations as bureaucratic and of bureaucracies as an extension of the power of the state. Thus they argued that bureaucracy would disappear with the 'withering away' of the state. Since the power of the state has barely diminished it is unlikely that we have less bureaucracy. However, Marx's work can be useful for us in thinking about how organising work for profit will systematically set up conflicts between those who will benefit and those who will lose out if pay and skills are minimised in the workforce. This is seen within the health workforce and in terms of health consequences for the general population.

Weber (1925) was concerned to look for reasons why modern Western capitalism had emerged. Traditionally, people had worked only to subsist, producing enough food or goods to cover their living needs. Capitalism requires people to work hard to make money and then use the money to make more money and to carry on working. People would only do this for powerful spiritual reasons. Weber claimed that the Protestant Reformation provided these reasons. The Lutherans altered the Catholic notion of **vocation** from a calling to leave the world in monastic retreat. Instead, they believed that God's purpose should be visibly fulfilled by working hard and efficiently at secular daily tasks. Work was a way demonstrably to forgo the pleasures of the flesh and, for Calvinists, also to demonstrate membership of the **elect** or the few chosen by God. It was in this way that hard work took on the kind of moral obligation it holds today.

Exercise

Analyse your current work motivation. Why have you opted to work in a health profession? Do you believe you have a vocation? If so, what are your work goals?

Weber's ideas can be useful in thinking about the different status given to different occupations and lifestyles, and the social motivations that affect health-related work choices. People assume that health professionals hold strong moral convictions about care and responsibility, but not all modern professionals surround their work with such an ethos.

Durkheim (1895) was concerned with how increasing speciali- sation in employment affected **social cohesion** – the forces which 'hold society together'. He investigated the impact of the growing **division of labour** on social solidarity. When there were few differences in the types of work people did, their experiences tended to be rather similar to one another, so society was cohesive because of these similarities. He called this **mechanical solidarity**. As industrialisation progressed and people started to perform many different and separate tasks in distinct work settings, it seemed surprising that, in spite of these differences, society remained, on the whole, cohesive. Durkheim argued that this was due to a form of **organic solidarity** in which we all became more dependent on one another because of the complexity of the industrial structure. Thus while the differences between us increased we became more interdependent. However, he suggested that all sorts of problems could arise in this situation. People might become more individualistic, less oriented towards the community and increasingly isolated in both work and home life.

Durkheim's work highlights how the mutual dependence between different parts of a social system can mean that a breakdown in any one area can have serious consequences throughout the rest of the system. It also raises the issue of how we can actually be said to be working together or to have a shared culture if we have very different working experiences and aims. Similarly, increased individualism raises doubts about the potential bases for community care.

Scientific management, human relations and cybernetics

Under the influence of Frederick W. Taylor (1911) in the early twentieth century there was a trend toward **scientific management**, which was concerned with enhancing the efficiency of work and of work organisations. Taylor held the view that it was in the interests of both management and workers to improve productivity. Management would be able to increase profits and workers to earn more if work was done efficiently. Physical movements in the workplace were meticulously timed and studied, accurately to link pay to production. Detailed research into organisational planning and decision-making aimed to produce practical recommendations which, when implemented, would help to minimise the inefficiencies of bureaucracies. This approach later developed into 'time and motion' studies.

Scientific management was criticised on the grounds that workers are neither solely motivated by pay, nor can be treated as if they work in isolation. The work of Elton Mayo (1933) established the foundations for a **human relations** tradition which tried to counteract the emphasis on efficiency at the expense of human needs. Mayo's research and a series of subsequent studies brought to light the importance of social relationships in the workplace and the influence on work of events in the broader society in which the work is conducted. Different types of work technology will influence the experience of work, as will technological change, differentials in company size and changes in company ownership.

By the 1960s work situations came to be analysed as forming part of a **complex socio-technical system**. Woodward (1965) showed how work technology, work organisation and the community context within which work was conducted are important influences on the labour process. Since the 1940s organisation analysts have also been interested in **cybernetics** – the study of how 'systems' work (see Open Systems Group 1981). The links to a functionalist theoretical perspective (see Chapter 1) are evident. Organisations could be studied as if they operated like machines or organisms with inputs and outputs. Work projects came to be managed systematically. The success of a project could depend upon the **critical path** to the production of goods and services – the most efficient and effective means for putting together the resources needed for doing a job. Productivity was regarded as a mechanical issue of timing input and output since these are measurable in terms of the accounting costs of products and services.

Once again this approach emphasised efficiency at the expense of the more human qualities of work. All of the management systems giving prime place to efficiency have encountered various forms of more or less organised **resistance**, including strikes. By the 1990s there had been a reaction to this and a revival of human relations influences in what is called **'soft systems'** analysis, in seminal work by Checkland (1981). In this way work organisation has to be studied as a cost-effective labour process, matched by an understanding of the social and psychological needs and aspirations of the workers.

Most of these traditions continue to influence current management practices to varying degrees. Even scientific management is still followed in some workplaces but is now known as 'work study engineering'.

Exercise

Consider your own work experiences. Which of these management practices have you been subjected to? What features of the work experience demonstrate the particular management perspective which was being applied?

Anyone who has worked on assembly lines, or where routine, repetitive tasks are to be performed, may have experienced attempts to measure the time taken to do a particular job. Some work organisations are more attuned to the social and emotional needs of their workers. Health care systems managers have been equally interested in applying this range of ideas to their organisations. We will look in more detail later at the consequences of each of these approaches in health work.

The changing structure of work

More recently, there have been fundamental changes in the global economy which have affected the experience of work for most people. The USA and Western Europe's world domination of industry and commerce has been overturned in favour of parts of East Asia. The decline in manufacturing industry has been partly offset by a growth in service industries and the increased professionalisation of certain occupations. However, service occupations have proven to be less durable and subject to rapid change depending on the fortunes of local economies. Braverman (1974) has argued that this **de-industrialisation** of the West has gone alongside a **deskilling** of labour – a breakdown of the components of the labour process into such small segments that ordinary workers have little understanding of their place in the total production scheme. He argues that much white collar work has become less skilled in this manner.

The global economy has become a corporate one dominated by a few large companies, so there has been a **narrowing of ownership**. A network of interlocking directorships with a few key financial institutions are responsible for the provision of major capital resources. A relatively small number of people control economies by co-operating with each other in the management of finance, prices and capital.

There is extensive debate, however, about just how much this economic control directly affects how we do our work. Many modern organisations have learned from the errors of scientific management and operate a form of **flexible management** which gives workers a lot more control over how they do their work. Since workers have little direct control over the larger economic structure, enhanced workplace control does little to guarantee the security of that work. Not many people have a sense of job security these days, either in terms of permanence or of being able to anticipate future work activity or work technology.

We may have a little more control over workplace experiences than people have had in the past. We all hold visions about an 'ideal' future which is related to more humane working conditions. We also know that there are practical limitations on such possibilities.

Exercise

Conduct your own 'vision workshop' about work.

To do this you need to consider what your 'ideal' work experience would be like. Take some time to outline the characteristics of the kind of work you would be really content to do. What tasks would it entail? What would the work setting be like? How would you like to be rewarded for it?

Consequences of the work process

The technologies of employment in factories – the assembly line in particular – have shaped obsessions with punctuality and with time in general. Office employment inherited many of these obsessions, backed by moral exhortations about the value of hard work and the avoidance of wasting time. Since we spend most of our lives working, our **occupation becomes a prime source of identity and social status**. Our place in society can be determined by our work. This is one way in which work orders society in terms of hierarchies of power and influence.

Workaholism can be one consequence of these obsessions. It is hard to stop work when it becomes a prime determinant of who we are. Our work setting may implicate us in particular networks of consensus or conflict. A **caring work ethos** makes it hard to engage in conflict, either with clients or employers, or with the state. Those employed in the production or distribution of goods may feel less inclined to allow themselves to be exploited for the sake of company profits.

Hierarchical work arrangements can accustom us to discipline and order, thereby helping to control the political system. More importantly, our position in a work hierarchy can have very direct consequences for our health. Marmot's (Marmot and Feeney 1996) study of civil servants showed that life expectancy increases for each increase in job grade. The higher the grade, the lower the risk of diabetes and heart disease.

Work is even linked to the education we seek or receive; as we discussed in Chapter 5 paid work has become the main goal of education. Ultimately, work may subordinate our identity to the demands of the job, such as when we take on a **sales personality**

or alter our behaviour in a way that is necessary for the job –
which may mean becoming something we are not.

Key questions

Do health care professionals have to cultivate a 'sales personality'? Is it necessary to put on a particular professional 'front' in
health care? If so, why? If not, why not? Look at what was
discussed about 'role' in Chapter 3.

Alienation

Such consequences of work are seen as detracting from our
opportunity to lead a full and rewarding life. Marx was the first to
apply the concept of **alienation** to the idea that work could be
dehumanising. Modern social science sees alienation as a multi-
dimensional concept, which helps in the analysis of the effects of
work on people. Seeman (1969) has identified its components as:

- **powerlessness** – feeling unable to control aspects of your life;
- **meaninglessness** – feeling unable to comprehend the
  purpose of your life;
- **isolation** – not feeling a part of broader social relationships;
- **self-estrangement** – feeling out of touch with yourself;
- **normlessness** – lacking commitment to shared social norms;
- **cultural estrangement** – feeling removed from established
  values.

Exercise

Using these dimensions, analyse some of your own work and
leisure situations. In what situations do you feel powerless or as
if there were no meaning to your actions? When analysing your

cont'd

Exercise

power, remember to look back at the political resources that you identified in Chapter 2. Go on to consider when you feel isolated, as if life has no meaning or you do not follow the same norms as others in your workplace, and so on.

Do this analysis for others with whom you regularly interact: colleagues, superiors, clients or friends.

The more of each of these dimensions we sense, the more alienated we are. Anyone holding all of these perceptions throughout all spheres of their life is really in a bad way. Most of us balance the more alienating parts of our life with those that give us meaning or a sense of belonging. Some of us may feel less alienated at home than during our time in paid employment; for example, we may feel more in control in our domestic environment. For others some of the more mundane tasks of housework can deprive them of a sense of freedom. Most of those tasks vary according to gender, and much housework is hidden in that it is taken for granted and rarely publicly acknowledged – thereby depriving those who do it of a sense of being valued or even of valuing themselves.

There has been much debate about how to make use of the concept of alienation in sociology. Fischer (1976) reviewed the arguments and showed how **job satisfaction** has to be seen as different from alienation. Those of us who are doing a job we enjoy or find rewarding may feel alienated due to a lack of power. In fact Seeman and Lewis (1995) showed that there are some very direct connections between a sense of powerlessness and ill health. Thus the concept of alienation may help us to understand those effects of employment which have special consequences for our health and whether some types of work and some forms of employment are better for our health than others. People often respond to the worst effects of alienation by avoiding work, taking more leisure or developing their own alternative resources or values within workplaces. Absenteeism, industrial 'accidents', industrial sabotage, fiddling and pilfering are among the responses taken by individuals, all of which may give rise to physical and/or mental health problems. People may also seek distractions at work such as listening to the radio or conversing with colleagues.

Key questions

What mechanisms have you employed, or seen others using, for dealing with alienation? For example, what have you done to gain more control in the workplace?

Collective action in work

The above responses are predominantly individual. Group responses to alienation are often more successful. Unionisation was once the main way in which workers could enhance the political and economic power of their occupational group. Trade and labour unions held a great deal of power when work was concentrated in a few major industries. Miners, dockworkers, power workers and transport workers were able to control work conditions and economic rewards by forming large organisations which could negotiate with government and employers. The decline of heavy industry, the growth of new industries and new occupations, and the implementation of legislation constraining union activity has effectively undermined the power of such groups. In the USA, for example, union membership declined from 40 per cent of the workforce in the 1950s to 15 per cent in the late 1990s.

Nonetheless, as Carpenter (1996) has pointed out, public service unions in the UK combined with user groups in the mid-1990s to resist government cost-cutting measures which would have led to a further deterioration of working conditions and a decline in service quality. This happened in major public utilities as well as within the health services.

Health workers have always had problems with the main union weapon – the withdrawal of labour – since it penalises the client more than the employer. The collective response which has been more popular in health care is **professionalisation**. Friedson (1994) discusses how professionalisation increases occupational power and enables more control of the workplace. When an occupation professionalises it takes on characteristics which mark it out from and enhances its social status in the community. Professionals have been held in esteem in the past because of the assumptions we make about their qualifications, educational level, specialist knowledge and dispassionate ability to act authoritatively in the best interests of a client. They have held an elite status.

Socialisation and training into a profession is often rigid and lengthy, so that members eventually share many values and are bound by a sense of identity. Professional status is long lasting, and ties between members are maintained by a common technical language and a clear status hierarchy. In the oldest professions the community – usually via its professional association – has a great deal of power over its members, in some cases regulating members' actions and practices as a substitute for state regulation. Ultimately, professional associations monopolise the availability of their practitioners' skills for the larger community by controlling entrance to the profession, the training of professionals and the assessment of skill levels. A skills monopoly usually enhances the price (fee) that can be charged for a service. Medicine, being nearly the oldest profession, does all of these things better than any other. For all these reasons professionalisation is one of the ways in which an occupation can resist the threat of alienation.

It is difficult to professionalise less visible work. Campaigns such as 'wages for housework' are attempts to have such work accorded its due recognition. Similarly, caring work has tended to be voluntary, unpaid, home-based, female work. It is therefore doubly ironic that the growth of professionalism has led to what Halmos (1970) called a **'personal service'** society.

Modern professionals have assumed a counselling ideology. They administer help through intimate physical and emotional relations; they show concern and sympathy for their client's problems. The essence of caring has become formalised. The ideal personal server shows compassion and insight, and employs both a 'scientific' method and empathy. Their underlying ideology is a socially determined belief system about the nature of human relationships.

Key questions

What might happen to informal care work as caring becomes more professionalised?

It is possible that the status of the informal carer may be lowered as more professionals get involved in caring. However, some of the lower formal caring roles are not being professionalised, although people might need evidence of having completed certain training qualifications in order to perform some caring tasks. In practice, given resource limitations, it is unlikely that much health care work will be done in the future without informal/voluntary helpers. Thus a changed relationship between formal and informal carers is likely.

Work in bureaucracies

Professionalisation alone cannot provide immunity from the complaints associated with alienation in work. Professionals' autonomy may be limited when they have to work in large, complex organisations. We spend most of our lives dealing with, working in or being dealt with by one formal organisation or another. **Formal organisations** are established in order to attain a specific goal or goals. Schools exist to educate, hospitals exist to return us to health – ideally.

Weber (1925) argued that there would be a growth in the most formal goal-oriented organisations – **bureaucracies** – as a result of the dominance of rational/legal forms of authority in the modern world (see Chapter 2). Bureaucracies involve integrated, clearly defined patterns of activity in which individuals gain authority, responsibilities and obligations according to the office they hold. There are ritualised ways of relating in bureaucracies which tend to emphasise impersonal procedures and which enhance the hierarchical statuses of officials. As a result power tends to be concentrated in the hands of those higher up the organisational structure; that is, bureaucracies tend towards **oligarchy**. Sociologists have been concerned with issues such as the effects of bureaucratic work on people's personalities, whether bureaucracies enhance or impede organisational efficiency and whether democratic, participatory decision-making is possible. The original goals for which organisations were set up are often not achieved; organisational goals may become **displaced** when officials grow too concerned with efficiency at the expense of the more human concerns of the organisation's employees and its clients.

> **Key questions**
>
> What formal organisations do you have to deal with?
>
> What sorts of problem do they confront you with?
>
> Do they inhibit the performance of your roles in any way?
>
> What can you do about that?

Whether a professional's autonomy is inhibited in a bureaucracy depends on several factors, including the size of the bureaucracy and the strength of the professional association involved. Thus, while nurses have long been recognised as professionals, they have, in the past, had little control over their conditions of work. This is partly due to the bureaucracy in large hospitals, rigid hierarchies in the profession and the relatively higher status of doctors.

Enhanced educational qualifications, changes in medical practice and organisation as well as changes in their own professional structure should all lead to an enhanced occupational status which could give nurses more control over their work situation. However, it may set them at odds with other nursing-related groups or may cause tensions within the profession between the different grades (Davies 1995).

In any case some of the predictions for the growth of ever-larger bureaucracies may be in doubt. The growth of privatised health care tends towards smaller organisations, and there is a lively debate among health economists about whether or not large hospitals produce efficiency gains.

Coping with change

Since change is a fundamental characteristic of modern society, the continued success of organisations will depend upon their ability to change. Contemporary organisations have to operate in a much more fluid, competitive, unstable environment. Contraction and restructuring are regular occurrences. Workforces are now better educated, with higher aspirations and expectations. Organisations can only survive and prosper if they exploit and reward the talents of such demanding human resources.

Hayes *et al.* (1988) argue that, to become responsive to change, organisations must learn how to learn: they must become **learning organisations**. Learning is inhibited by defensive strategies adopted by participants at all levels in the organisation. Defensive routines emerge as a consequence of misunderstandings and protectionist processes. Modern organisation analysts argue that learning can only occur if the talents of all throughout the organisation are exploited through smaller work teams. In the past even large formal organisations could operate effectively if they had strong, clear leadership and an authority structure fitting the organisation's goals. Modern organisations are rarely structured in a simple pyramidal hierarchy. More often they are based on a devolved, teamworking system which aims to foster **synergy**. Synergy works on the principle that the whole is greater than the sum of the parts. Something more emerges from the team working together than from the individual skills or qualities.

It is argued that the essential qualities of good teamwork include: a clear agreed objective; distinct and firm roles for all members of the team; dispensability (the team could continue without you); and trust between team members. For this to work the team has to be of manageable size, ideally between ten and fifteen members. Anything larger and some of the classic **dysfunctions** of formal/bureaucratic organisations will begin to operate: fragmentation, reduced trust, unintended outcomes and the displacement of goals.

Exercise

Look at any team you have worked in.

Which of the above criteria applied?

How did this affect the successful achievement of the team's aims?

Many companies have introduced smaller working teams in recent years. This has meant quite a change from the mass production line for motor cars first advocated by Henry Ford for a less educated, more regimented workforce. **Post-Fordist** workers expect much more engagement with their work, identify more closely with their immediate work group and take on stronger collective responsibilities for what they produce.

Learning organisations will respect the views of all workers, often beginning with those at grass roots level, since they are often the first to recognise flaws in systems or products. Success is not always guaranteed, so teams must be given the opportunity to try things out and fail, without too heavy a penalty being incurred.

Being indispensable does not mean that all roles are interchangeable, and many theorists have pointed to the importance of clarity and firmness in the maintenance of team roles. The most influential work in this area has been by Meredith Belbin (1981). Certain work roles have to be performed by some member of the team. By placing people in the role to which they are most suited it may be possible to establish effective teamworking more rapidly:

- The **plant** is creative, imaginative, unorthodox and solves difficult problems, but might not be good with ordinary people.

- The **co-ordinator** is mature, confident, trusting and makes a good chairperson in clarifying goals and promoting decision-making.

- The **shaper** is dynamic, outgoing and can find ways round obstacles, but might be temperamental.

- The **teamworker** is sociable, attentive and perceptive, can find ways of accommodating others, can thus build teams while avoiding friction, but may be indecisive under pressure.

- The **completer** is painstaking, conscientious and produces the goods on time, but may worry and be reluctant to delegate.

- The **implementer** is disciplined, reliable and efficient and can turn ideas into actions, but may be a little conservative and inflexible.

- The **resource investigator** is an extrovert, enthusiastic and communicative explorer of opportunities, but may lose interest after initial bursts of enthusiasm.

- The **specialist** is single-minded, self-starting and dedicated, bringing valued knowledge or skills, while being restricted to a specialism.

- The **monitor evaluator** is sober, strategic, discerning of all options and can make sound judgements, but may lack drive and the ability to inspire others.

> **Exercise**
>
> Do you recognise yourself, or any of your colleagues, in these roles?
>
> Does any one in particular apply to you or them, or do your talents embrace more than one role?

Healthy organisations

It seems that the health, and thus the success, of an organisation depends on its ability to learn, to place employees in appropriate organisational tasks and to care about them. This means that learning organisations should also be **caring organisations**. Such organisations must possess an affiliative or a warmly supportive attitude to all those with whom they deal. There must be respect for the individuality and tolerance of the kind of difference which encourages innovation. Honest, open communication is vital, as is a balance between freedom and order. Spontaneity and fun in the company of others is also important. Since people spend so much time in work, it must remain enjoyable; thus play and games in the workplace must be allowed. Finally, there must be some kind of overarching system of values and beliefs which defines collective goals and which permits members to cope with loss and change, which are inevitable features of organisational life.

> **Exercise**
>
> Look at the organisations or teams you have previously analysed. How many of these latter features do they possess?

There are times when organisations cannot be too adventurous. Running through all these 'healthy' qualities is the need to combine or balance two opposing principles: the freedom to allow independence, spontaneity and creativity, and the discipline of an ordered hierarchy in which the potential for chaos is limited and individuals can feel some degree of security.

Boundaries and clear identification of work skills, training and tasks are important in establishing the status claims of particular types of working group. This may explain, at least in part, why groups that are seen as doing work that is less demonstrably skilled, such as caring work, may be less valued and less visible than if they were doing 'real work'. If nurses, for example, are unable to establish the effectiveness of the care which they provide, they may find it difficult to establish their claims to higher professional status. Occupational therapy is similarly vulnerable to forces that diminish its economic and political position in the health care market unless it can establish a robust knowledge base. Such knowledge must detail the health-promoting qualities of particular elements of the experience of work.

Structural change in work patterns

There has always been a higher proportion of part-time women employees in nursing and health care work. This is becoming the typical pattern of work in advanced industrial economies. Men are retiring earlier and their job opportunities have declined sharply while those for women have grown. Many large employers have cut back on full-time jobs in favour of part-time, short-contract work. There are likely to be far fewer, full-time, lifelong career occupations and more frequent job changes. Occupational insecurity is high, with the proportion of full-time tenured employees in the adult working population substantially decreased.

The Fordist assembly line is disappearing. Fordism entailed many low-skilled, low-paid jobs, each worker contributing a small part to a production process geared to a mass market. The Post-Fordist view is that, because people no longer want exactly the same things as their neighbours, the market has now become highly differentiated. New technology enables and requires increased flexibility in production. Current demand is for **niche marketing**, by which goods and services are produced for targeted groups of consumers. This will require even more flexibility in the worker. Only a small-core permanent workforce will be needed, which can be supported by a more **flexible peripheral workforce** able to meet short-term demands. Labour adjustments can be made according to rapid changes in the market. These trends are intensified by emphases on customer satisfaction and cost effectiveness, requiring changes to meet ever more varied demands.

Charles Handy (1989) suggests that **portfolio working** or episodic participation in employment could become the norm. Lifelong retraining and reskilling would be essential to the maintenance of a portfolio of relevant skills. Many smaller, private employers are unlikely to take on the costs of update training needed to maintain standards, so the burden would be placed on individuals to learn in their own time using information technology and distance learning. One possible advantage could be a higher status for both part-time work and informal care work. This might even lead to accreditation for working experiences in families or in voluntary activity outside formal employment, or it may simply lead to ever-widening gaps between groups with substantially different incomes and employment conditions.

Handy also points to the growth of **virtual organisations** – where work is conducted via information technology, removing the need for a physical office building which is attended daily by the workers. They can work at home and at large distances, communicating via the Internet.

This more flexible workforce includes professionals who desire change and are liable to be bored by monotonous and repetitive work, but putting new organisational and occupational structures together is bound to create tensions and conflicts. A problem of professional work boundaries is inevitable. Professional change brings changes in responsibility, authority, tasks performed, teamwork relationships, conflict with management and inter-professional disputes over occupational boundaries.

Change in occupational structure for health professionals

Walby and Greenwell (1994) show how such processes have, necessarily, influenced occupations involved in the delivery of public health care. Conflict is not the inevitable outcome of tensions between professionals, but traditional working practices and former professional alliances will change. The balance between care, treatment and relationships with patients is particularly contested in the boundary between medicine and nursing. Junior doctors' roles may be threatened by the extension of nurses' roles. The growth of specialisms in radiography raises questions about the radiologist's role. Physiotherapists may have to change practices as chiropractic and osteopathy gain legitimacy.

A major area of conflict is between doctors and managers. Managers drive to improve bed occupancy rates, control ward budgets and increase patient throughput. The line of accountability becomes obscured by the distinction between clinical and administrative demands. Devolution of financial accountability takes decision-making and the prioritising of health targets down to the patient level, giving rise to even greater tensions in the workplace. More disputes over who controls treatment, task priorities and mundane duties such as cleaning and tidying are inevitable.

The working patterns of nurses and doctors have always differed despite the need for them to engage in teamwork. Nurses are tied to wards and fixed shifts and breaks. Doctors move between wards, are on call and can take breaks regardless of time. The two professions traditionally bear different relationships to the major management theories. Nursing has been dominated by principles of scientific management, while medicine has always had a structure more likely to fit into soft systems theory.

Conclusion

Work and employment are clearly important to people. The nature and organisation of work is a fundamental determinant of adult experience in society. It affects the life chances of people and their families as well as where and how they live.

At least one health profession – occupational therapy – has the primary goal of returning persons with disabilities to useful occupation within society. The core of their professional ethos is the belief that occupation is a vital adaptive medium and engagement in occupation can favourably influence health and display respect for the person. There are side-effects of work which can be supportive to health but which have little to do with the job content. Thus playing and joking with work colleagues, the community of work relationships or escape from domestic pressures can all have therapeutic effects.

We have stressed how the organisation, status and resources offered by different kinds of work can cause specific problems for physical and psychological health. Cary Cooper, an organisational psychologist, has pointed out how the 'enterprise culture' of the 1980s in the UK produced further obsessions with working long hours in stressful conditions, which severely damaged individual health and family life (Cooper 1996). Professional health carers, too, face these problems. The structure, the technology and the conditions of their work can similarly cause alienation. Professionalisation enhances autonomy and can insulate against some of the problems of health care, but even this may not be resistant to the demands of modern management and changes in the organisation of work.

Evidence of the links between specific job-related illness and disease, bad health practices and health outside work and in old age is overwhelming. It is not that lower-class groups, women or ethnic groups place a lower value on health, but their working conditions, household resources and lack of contact with or knowledge of the health system are closely related to decisions or actions in relation to health. In the next chapter we consider in detail the underlying social causes of inequality which have consequences for the seeking and maintenance of health.

Further reading

Argyris, C. (1993) *Knowledge for Action (A Guide to Overcoming Barriers to Organizational Change)*, San Francisco: Jossey-Bass.
A key practical text which identifies structural factors in resistance to change.

Jolley, M. and Allan, P. (1989) 'The professionalisation of nursing: the uncertain path', Chapter 1 in *Current Issues in Nursing*, London: Chapman & Hall.
Summarises most of the relevant issues.

Kanter, R.M. (1983) *The Change Masters: Corporate Entrepreneurs at Work*, London: Unwin.
A readable series of case studies which can be applied to health care work.

Sims, D., Fineman, S. and Gabriel, Y. (1993) *Organizing and Organizations*, London: Sage.
A comprehensive and accessible text on organisations and bureaucracy.

Vault, M.L. de (1991) *Feeding the Family: The Social Organisation of Caring as Gendered Work*, Chicago: University of Chicago Press.
Aptly illustrates the invisible nature of women's household work obligations.

Chapter 7 Equal and Unequal Opportunities

In most societies some groups of people have more access to material resources, to health and to respect than others. Most health and care resources are taken up in dealing with disadvantaged groups. As we have indicated inequality and the lack of political resources to remedy inequalities are central to meeting health care needs.

Inequality and difference

One of the many paradoxes of human experience is that we are, at the same time, similar but different. We share the fact that we are mortal human beings. This makes us all **equal** in one respect, but we are also unique. Each of us inhabits our own particular place in space and time. Only *I* have had my experiences and inherited my physical characteristics. Only *you* have had and inherited yours. However, we find it hard to handle complete difference or complete sameness. We like to think that some people are similar to us and some are different from us, and we organise our world according to those characteristics.

In most societies people do not see each other as equals. To differentiate between their fellow creatures all human societies use criteria which are of importance in that society. Societies have **different priorities** over the things that are **valued**.

The most common criterion for differentiating people is **gender**. People generally treat other people differently according to their sex because sex is something that matters to us. For the purpose of selecting a mate, reproduction or the pleasure of company, it is important that we can tell the difference between men and women. However, for most of human history females have been regarded as physically and intellectually inferior to males and have consequently not been treated equally.

Another difference is **ethnicity**. We treat people differently according to their skin colour, clothing or behaviour. Ethnicity matters because we need to know the correct way to greet people, whether they intend to be friendly or hostile, or whether they are in any way similar to ourselves or might engage in behaviour which we may not like. There are many historical and cultural reasons for this behaviour, one having to do with the way in which both gender and ethnicity are linked to other **scarce** and **valued resources** in society.

Most societies value people's achievements in terms of **wealth**, social **prestige** or specialist **skills**. As we discussed in Chapter 2, all societies distinguish individuals in terms of the power they possess. If everyone possessed an equal amount of these valued resources, social inequality would not exist. However, these resources are distributed unevenly. By highlighting differences between people which are seen as vital to a society, we begin to point to **patterns of inequality** within that society.

Inequality becomes patterned or structured when individuals are **classified** together with others who match them on these key criteria. They then share similar characteristics with those others and, as a result, similar access to the unevenly distributed and valued resources. People and groups are then often **evaluated** according to how they have been classified with others, so one group is seen as better than or superior to another. For example, one group may be wealthier (using economic criteria), more powerful (using political criteria) or more honourable (using social status criteria) than another.

Thus women in most societies have been accorded fewer of these resources and therefore a lower status. The same has happened to ethnic groups which are in the minority in a society. In general, people have been seen as belonging to different **social classes** according to some combination of their economic position, their power and/or their status. Some socialist feminists have argued that women can be seen to form a separate social class to men in these respects.

Given that this evaluation is carried out according to valued resources, groups tend to be viewed hierarchically, as above or below each other. Society can be seen as arranged like layers of rock strata, which is why sociologists use the term **social stratification** to describe the pattern or structure of social inequality.

Exercise

What criteria do you use to evaluate different groups of people?

Consider the following list of valued resources: physical strength; physical fitness; language skills; intellectual ability; physical appearance... add to the list other resources which you consider valuable. Remember the resources list in Chapter 2.

How are such resources variously allocated to groups in terms of gender, class, age or ethnicity?

Understanding inequality is particularly vital to explaining the uneven distribution of health resources. Differences in valued priorities play a part in decisions about allocating scarce health resources and in rewarding different kinds of health care work. For example, the structure of health occupations frequently reflects gender inequality. Patterns of wealth, status and power are reflected in the delivery of health services. As a consequence people differ in their access to healthy lifestyles, the resources to maintain health and the control of health-related services.

Measuring social inequality

To understand how a system of social stratification works we have to investigate its **objective** and its **subjective** features: how the system looks from both the point of view of an independent outside observer as well as from insiders' views and experiences of their place within the system. Objective features may not necessarily be more accurate, but they are easier to measure. Thus, in order to demonstrate that some social groups are less advantaged than others, sociologists will use **occupation** and **income** as **indicators** of differences in access to valued resources between social groups. Such information is relatively easy to obtain and offers a fair degree of accuracy. Ordinarily, we use the way in which people speak as a subjective criterion of their position in a social hierarchy. This is harder to measure precisely, but subjective experiences of the 'goodness' or 'badness', 'rightness' or 'wrongness', of inequality may be central to how far people support an unequal system, transmit it or enforce it in daily life.

Subjective measures of inequality

'**Social status**' is the phrase often used to refer to the subjective estimates of a person's position in a social hierarchy. Prestige can be seen as separate from formal positions in a hierarchy. Thus being able to sing well may be important in social circles, but it holds little value in a commercial organisation where budget-balancing skills such as accountancy are more useful. Status varies according to the settings in which social judgements are made.

A hierarchical status system is built out of the judgements of members of a society about the standing or rank of individuals, groups and/or families with respect to one another. Such judgements are often made visible by the use of signs or symbols of deference and respect.

In modern industrial societies there are two major **indicators of status**:

1. **Occupation** is probably the main determinant of prestige in most societies because occupations take up most of our time; they provide income, social esteem and power, and there are clear occupational differences in skill, responsibility and authority. There are also varying requirements in the levels of education and training required for different occupations.

2. **Lifestyle** also becomes a sign of rank and is indicated by, for example, work hours, time off work, clothing, manners, newspapers and books read, place and type of residence and membership of certain organisations. Lifestyle remains linked to occupation.

Social status has important consequences quite apart from any economic resources on which it is based. We treat people differently according to our perception of their social worth.

Different patterns of consumption are linked to economic resources and these, in turn, affect prestige. For example, one can have the manners and accent of the elite, but without the supporting income it would be difficult to maintain the high-status lifestyle.

Exercise

To understand how status affects individuals, try answering the following questions:

Whom do you most admire?...and why?

Whom do you most respect?...and why?

Whom do you most envy?...and why?

Do you have a hero or heroine?...why do you hold them in such esteem?

What do such people possess that you don't?

What do such people possess that you too would like to have?

Compare your estimations of status with those held by your friends or colleagues. Note the similarities and differences. These will highlight similarities or difference in community member-ship or personal experience.

There cannot be an integrated social status system for a whole society unless people commonly agree on the criteria by which prestige or access to valued resources is granted to particular groups. The current debates about employment rights for the disabled offer an illustration of the dilemmas involved. Thornton and Lunt (1995) point out how disabled people are at a structural disadvantage in terms of both the quantity and the quality of employment available to them. There has been a decline in policies which oblige employers to take on disabled people. Treating access to employment as a right, for any group, maintains its inequitable distribution. Disability groups advocate a movement towards independent living which places an onus on disabled people to take control of their own lives. In other words, the disabled want to be accorded the same status as

other people in society rather than treated as special because of
their disability.

Key questions

With reference to your own experience of workplaces, which
groups and which people are accorded high status and why?

Objective indicators of inequality

In order to study social inequality objectively, groups of people
have to be assigned to categories according to their society's
priorities. An individual's position in the economic market for
labour or property – their social class position – is best indicated
by their occupation. It may not indicate all aspects of inequality,
but it is convenient in that most people are willing to give basic
information about their occupation.

A variety of occupational scales have been used throughout
the twentieth century. Early scales were basic, containing an
upper, middle and lower classification. As changes took place in
the number, nature and distribution of occupations over time,
the scales became increasingly sophisticated. Objective indicators will change as the structured inequalities they measure
become more complex.

The range of scales used are outlined in most of the major
introductory sociology texts (see, for example, Haralambos and
Holborn 1991, Chapter 2). The UK Office of Population
Censuses and Surveys conducted an overhaul of the classification system in the late 1980s, occupations now being grouped
according to a Standard Occupational Classification (SOC)
(Table 7.1 overleaf).

Table 7.1　Standard Occupational Classification

Major groups:	Examples of occupations	Estimated nos. (1992)	SOC code no.
1. Managers and Administrators	Managers and proprietors in service industries Farm owners and managers	751,610 200,150	179 160
2. Professional Occupations	Engineers and technologists Higher and further education teachers	441,710 150,400	21 231
3. Associate Professional and Technical Occupations	Scientific technicians Computer analysts/ programmers Nurses	303,390 145,300 484,320	30 32 340
4. Clerical and Secretarial Occupations	Secretaries/typists (general) Clerks (general)	827,310 646,590	45 430
5. Craft and Related Occupations	Carpenters and joiners Electricians	309,400 248,110	570 521
6. Personal and Protective Service Occupations	Child care and related occupations Health and related occupations (care assistant level)	313,410 514,680	65 64
7. Sales Occupations	Sales assistants/ check-out operators Sales representatives	1,180,560 379,260	72 71
8. Plant and Machine Operatives	Packers, bottlers, canners, fillers Chemicals/process operatives	247,190 205,460	862 82
9. Other Occupations	Cleaners, domestics Counterhands, catering assistants	778,600 209,790	958 953

Source: Data drawn from OPCS, Economic Activity, Volume 1, June 1994.

Indices of occupation say something about an individual's status, power, influence and life chances. Other objective indices of inequality are either difficult to define or prove difficult for researchers to extract. Income and wealth, for example, appear to be easily quantifiable in monetary terms, but accurate information on both is difficult to obtain.

Distribution of wealth

There are two main problems with assessing the distribution of wealth in any society. First, wealth is difficult to define and therefore hard to measure. It cannot simply be equated with income, since anyone who spends more than they earn – no matter how much it is – would not be wealthy. Wealth is assumed to include things such as how much one has in a bank account, owned property, assets, stocks and shares held in companies and so on. Second, people do not willingly reveal their income to researchers or to government officials and, even if they do, certain items may be forgotten, ignored or avoided. Assets held in foreign bank deposits may never be revealed. In spite of these measurement difficulties, however one measures it, it is quite clear that a relatively small minority of the population have always owned the majority of private wealth.

After the world-wide economic recession of the 1930s there was a growth of state welfare policies in most developed industrial countries and a slow but steady redistribution of wealth towards poorer families and households. The 1980s in the UK and USA saw the first reversal of this trend of lessening differentials between rich and poor in thirty years. In 1996 a United Nations Report on Human Development announced that the **total wealth of the 358 wealthiest people in the world was equal to the combined incomes of the poorest 45 per cent of the world's people**, that is, 2.3 billion people. Developing countries have 80 per cent of the world's population but only 22 per cent of the world's total wealth.

Whatever criteria are used to measure wealth, it is reasonable to assume that the publicly available information will underestimate the extent of the inequality of wealth distribution. It remains within the interests and resources of those with the greatest wealth to disguise and minimise the extent of their wealth. While the possession of wealth is a factual indicator of social inequality, this, by itself, does not determine the relationship between this form of economic inequality and inequalities in status and power. In any society we would have to examine the restrictions imposed upon the use of personal wealth. What discretion to dispose of their wealth do individuals have? What difference do such inequalities in the distribution of wealth have on people's lifestyles and life chances? How does it affect their health opportunities? Does the possession of most of the wealth by a few prevent the poorer groups in society from enhancing their own life chances? Only then can we understand the full social and political consequences of an unequal distribution of wealth.

Key questions

One way of understanding these implications is to ask these questions of yourself. What difference would a sudden increase in your own personal wealth make to your lifestyle? How would it affect your health? What do wealthy people do with their wealth?

Wealth can lead to extremely healthy or unhealthy practices. Opportunities for healthy activity do not depend upon economic resources alone. Lifestyle practices are cultural choices which may take little account of health (see Chapter 13).

Poverty

At the other extreme of the unequal distribution of economic resources are the poor. Here, the distinction raised earlier between the subjective and the objective perspective on inequality is vital. There can be a mismatch between the **subjective meaning** of inequality for a person and the **objective measure** of that person's position on an independent hierarchical scale. Thus a sociologist might use income or occupation as an index of someone's position in a hierarchy, but this might not match the individual's evaluation of their own position in that hierarchy. For example, a sociologist with information about income differentials in society may place someone in a low-income group on a scale indicating the distribution of incomes. That person, however, may be unaware of how high some incomes are in their society and may consider themselves to be well paid, since they lack accurate information with which to make comparisons.

Similarly, some people judge themselves not to be in poverty since they have all they expect to have or all they feel they need. Clearly, both the objective and the subjective meanings of inequality are vital to a full understanding of the effects of inequality since, even though people in poverty do not see themselves as poor, the objective problem of poverty remains for society, so much so that we can see the consequences of such poverty all around us and social policy action may be required.

In order to take action to address the problem it is first necessary to assess how much of a problem it is and to be able to identify which particular individuals and groups are suffering. Only by attempting such objective measures can we compile evidence to demonstrate the extent of social inequalities in the social structure and what their consequences are for life and health chances.

Objective measures of poverty

There are problems for developing an objective definition of 'absolute' poverty. Charles Booth (1889) was the first to point out that poverty can only be defined in relation to a generally accepted standard of living in a specific society at a particular time in its history. In such terms poverty means **lacking the resources needed to survive and to take part in the life of the community**.

Attempts have been made to measure poverty objectively since the later nineteenth century. Measures have been based on criteria such as income, food, housing and clothing, things which are physically necessary for survival. In this sense minimum requirements are seen as **absolute**, necessities without which people are unable to live. Subsistence becomes the extreme measure of poverty.

Whether subsistence is adequate still depends on the societal context in which we operate. It can be argued that people are in poverty when they have the lowest standards of living for their society over a long enough period to undermine the health, morale and self-respect of an individual or group. This represents a standard of living so low as to exclude people from the life of their community. For this reason Seebohm Rowntree (1899) introduced the notion of a **poverty line** – the minimum weekly sum necessary to keep a family healthy. Poverty could then be measured as an attribute of the poorest 'x' per cent of the population – the percentage of families falling below the poverty line. In this way societies are compared with each other in terms of how well they deal with extremes of inequality. Even though a list of what is needed for subsistence varies between societies and communities, it has to include items which are regarded as essential. These include a normal diet, adequate clothing, the means to participate in social activities, access to amenities and standards of acceptable accommodation.

Exercise

What items are considered necessary for survival in your society?

If you were poor, what would be your minimum requirements for survival?

What sort of food... and how much of it?

What sort of housing or shelter?

What sort of clothing... and how much of it?

Would you expect any leisure or recreational items?.... What kinds?

How far would these items meet minimum health requirements?

Do you think your list would be acceptable to people who are actually poor in your society?

Would others who are not poor in your society agree with your list? – Ask them.

It is, however, surprising how much disagreement there is, even within the same society, about how much of which items are considered essential for survival and how much the poor could be allowed in order to make living worthwhile.

Recent poverty scales for industrial societies have included many of the following items:

● **Clothing** for each person – a warm waterproof coat; two pairs of shoes; a change of clothes.

● **Food** – at least one substantial meal each day; meat and/or fish every other day; some fresh fruit and vegetables.

● **Housing** – a damp-free home that has heating for living areas when the weather is cold; an indoor toilet, bath or shower not shared with another household; beds for everyone in the household; some carpeted rooms in living areas; separate bedrooms (for the different sexes over the age of ten).

- **Leisure and amenities** – adequate public transport for access to shopping, schooling and work; an annual holiday; toys and other leisure/sports equipment for children; enough money for a hobby, the occasional night out, some cigarettes and some alcohol; a garden.
- **Household consumer durables** – a refrigerator; a washing machine; a telephone; a television; a radio/music centre; a car if public transport is inadequate.

Key questions

How many of these items were on your list? Are there any things on this list that you think ought not to be there? If not, why not?

Many people in advanced industrial societies do not have some of these items. Poverty of this sort is a condition in which individuals and families are deprived of the opportunities, comforts and means for self-respect which the majority of people in their society enjoy. Yet, compared with some groups in other societies, they could be considered well off. Thus people in slum houses in Europe and America are regarded as poor by comparison with others in their society. In some third world countries they would be regarded as rich since they do, at least, have a house.

Social policy which is aimed at reducing extremes of inequality and to some extent redistributing the balance of wealth depends upon attempts to measure poverty objectively using such lists and income measures based on the costs of purchasing such items. However, even such apparently objective measures can be altered. In 1988 the UK government changed the methods for measuring income. They adopted a method for averaging incomes across households, which prevented adequate comparisons over time (that is, with previous statistics on poverty), thus making it impossible to compare the effects of successive governments' policies. There are now no ways of comparing changes in real incomes with rates of welfare benefits actually paid in the UK. This also makes it difficult to collect statistics comparing how different countries deal with poverty.

In order to try to establish some comparative measures, the European Union (EU) used a Households Below Average Income statistic (HBAI) as a measure of poverty. Using this estimate an extra 4 million children in the USA fell into poverty during the 1980s, even though the wealth generated by the country's economy grew by one-fifth. In the EU the number of people living in poverty grew from 38 million to 52 million between 1975 and 1988. In the UK those living in poverty rose from 5 million in 1979 to 14.1 million in 1993. During this period the living standards of rich and poor moved wider apart, and the poorest tenth of the population experienced a fall in their real income of 18 per cent compared with the average rise of 37 per cent for the population as a whole.

International organisations have approached poverty by attempting to establish uniform minimum human rights which would give people access to the minimum resources needed to live a reasonable life. These are specified in the Universal Declaration of Human Rights (1948), the International Covenant of Civil and Political Rights (1966) and the International Covenant of Economic, Social and Cultural Rights (1966). They include rights to health care, education, enough to eat, a home, a livelihood, clean water, a sustainable environment, equality of opportunity, protection from violence and a say in the future.

Key questions

Which of these rights were on your earlier list?

All this shows that even the objective measurement of poverty is **relative** to the general standard of living in the society, the distribution of wealth, the status system and social expectations.

Subjective perceptions of poverty: wants, needs and relative deprivation

Subjective perceptions of inequality are more relative than objective measures. One problem is the distinction between **wants** and **needs**. Subsistence measures assume that people know what they need to survive. In extremes of poverty this is certainly the case. We know when we are hungry and cold and need food and shelter.

When basic needs are adequately satisfied we tend to focus on wants, but we do not always know what we need. For example, in order to achieve certain desired occupational goals we may need particular kinds of knowledge or contacts, and we may not know this. Alternatively, without adequate knowledge of nutrition we might want things that are tasty but which do not meet our nutritional needs.

Key questions

How can we tell the difference between wants and needs?

Who has the right to say that our wants are not really needs?

Are there things which you feel you 'need' which others might regard as 'wants'?

Have you seen people seeking 'needs' which you feel are 'wants'?

Which of the items in your subsistence list above do you think can be seen by others as something you want but do not need?

In terms of poverty the question is, first, whether or not people perceive themselves as poor, and second, whether they regard that as unfair, resent it and act to remedy it. The concept illustrating this most forcefully is that of **relative deprivation**, which was explored in some detail by W.G. Runciman (1972). He explains how you can only be relatively deprived of something you do not have but think you should and could have. Even wealthy people can experience this. If you have an expensive car, and one of your neighbours who seems to have a similar job, lifestyle and income has an even more expensive one, you may resent it and seek to buy one yourself – thereby 'keeping up with the Joneses'.

On the other hand, if you are deprived of something and do not perceive others in the same position as yourself as having that thing, you may not expect it nor do anything about attaining it. Your neighbours could be drinking champagne daily, but unless they invite you to join them, or you catch sight of the empty bottles, you will be none the wiser so not experience relative deprivation. Thus the poor may not feel relatively deprived if they do not see it as feasible to expect some of the material and healthy living resources which others enjoy.

For such reasons Peter Townsend (1970) has argued that the attempt to draw a distinction between **absolute** and **relative** poverty is misleading. All inequality is relative, the question is relative to what? Who measures this and how do they do the measuring? Finally, what is done with the information once gained? It can be used to redress the balance of inequality either by altering people's perceptions or by improving the access of the poor to the resources of which they are deprived. Townsend's own 'deprivation index' moved beyond subsistence to include items which people could reasonably expect to achieve and of which they were relatively deprived – such as annual holidays. Using this index he estimated more than 20 per cent of the UK population to be in poverty in 1968/69. Those who challenged Townsend's data did so on the grounds that relative deprivation cannot be included in objective measures of poverty.

However measured, all the recent evidence suggests that world-wide poverty is on the increase. The United Nations Human Development Report (1996) claimed that, in seventy countries, people are on average poorer than they were in 1980. Between 1960 and 1991 the richest 20 per cent of the world's population increased their share of the world's wealth from 70 per cent to 85 per cent. The wealth of the poorest 20 per cent fell from 2.3 per cent to 1.4 per cent. By 1991 85 per cent of the world's population was receiving only 15 per cent of the world's income. Real extremes of deprivation are seen when regions in the world suffer famine. This happens even when there are gluts of some foods in other parts of the world, suggesting a global economic system unable to redress the extremes of inequality. Interestingly, those countries in South East Asia and the East which have seen the greatest economic growth have been the fairest in the division of income and assets and have had greatest success in keeping unemployment down.

The culture of poverty

Most people are aware of the cumulative nature of the problem of inequality and poverty. Acquiring more wealth appears to be easier if you already have some. Many commentators have shown how **social disadvantage is cumulative**. Some combinations of conditions for impoverishment may create vicious circles, driving people into an inescapable state of poverty. The education system works better for groups higher up the social hierarchy than for those lower down. Welfare benefits systems often penalise lower-paid workers, stopping them from improving themselves by setting inappropriate income thresholds. Lacking the means to maintain certain basic minimum standards is also cumulative in terms of people's health, with a deteriorating ability to meet basic physical needs: to provide warmth, housing, nutrition and to satisfy ambitions or expectations of a less stressful life.

More recently, research suggests that if people cannot escape the condition of poverty, an **underclass** of highly impoverished people may be created, existing on the margins of society and ignored by governments and the more respectable members of society. William Wilson (1978) suggests that this has happened to African Americans in the USA. While blacks are distributed throughout the American class structure, some are trapped in urban ghettos in such a cycle of cumulative disadvantage. The conservative writer Charles Murray (1984, 1990) believes welfare dependency to be the main reason for the existence of such an underclass, which is not confined to any one ethnic group and is growing in size in the UK.

Key questions

Do you agree that there is such an underclass?

What categories of people tend to get trapped in such conditions? How do we identify them? In other words, what evidence is there for the existence of such a class? What status or esteem do they hold? How do they gain access to any resources?

Some modern governments encourage the workforce to be more flexible by taking non-permanent jobs for less pay, but social security systems do not accommodate this since taking temporary jobs interferes with bureaucratic routines. Such a system encourages people to find small amounts of work and then keep it secret, even if they are normally honest. Thus the system either encourages dishonesty or discourages people from working at all.

The idea that a culture of poverty becomes self-perpetuating within families and within particular localities was first outlined by Oscar Lewis (1961), who suggested that people become resigned to a situation of disadvantage and devise ways of living with it. Their values, norms and standards produce and maintain poverty. They seldom take opportunities which would allow them to change their circumstances. Children grow up in such a culture, taking on their parents' attitudes and behaviour, and poverty thus continues from one generation to the next. The subculture of the poor is characterised by narrow perspectives on the world, restrictions in the immediate environment and feelings of marginality, helplessness, dependence, inferiority and resignation. Such views prevent an escape from poverty and suggest that people who are poor are inherently different from the remainder of society. It is in this way that a vicious circle is created which perpetuates certain cultural patterns.

One problem with this approach is the suggestion that the cultural patterns of the poor are the cause of their poverty. It is used by those who wish to blame the poor for their own poverty, and it implies that if only the poor would change their values, poverty would disappear. The concept is convenient for those in government who wish to reduce social security costs by cutting welfare benefits to make the poor 'stand on their own two feet'. The alternative, they claim, is welfarism, which creates a nation of weak, benefit-dependent people.

The culture of poverty certainly exists and it may well be caused by poverty, but it should not be seen as a *cause of* poverty. The development of a **subculture of poverty** – a culture within a culture – establishes values and ways of behaving which help the poor to cope with being poor. It may be that one consequence of this subculture is to encourage habits and practices which keep them poor and trapped within their culture. In most other respects, the poor are like the rest of society, with similar aspirations only with less money and less opportunity to get it.

The poor are often ghettoised for practical reasons to do with meeting basic requirements. Low-cost housing and cheap supermarkets tend to be located in the same area. Thus people will be stigmatised by where they live and the sorts of consumer goods they buy, making it harder to associate with those outside that way of life.

Poverty and health

For such reasons research has linked material poverty both directly and indirectly to poor health and poor physical development. Health deficiencies arise among the poor because of their economic and cultural inability to realise a healthier lifestyle (Townsend and Davidson 1982, Whitehead 1987).

Without sufficient money people are unable to provide themselves and their families with adequate housing, nutrition, clothing and heating. Levels of hygiene may be lower. Alcoholism and smoking are more prevalent as relatively cheap and accessible forms of recreation. Health problems such as respiratory infections are caused by damp and lack of heating; poor diet reduces resilience to infections and increases the incidence of disease. An unsafe environment leads to accidents. Illnesses associated with overcrowding and poor sanitation are also more prevalent in areas with a high incidence of poverty. People who live in poverty are less likely to have the means to travel to clinics and hospitals, which means that they are less likely to attend antenatal appointments or take advantage of health screening opportunities. A lack of transport also means having to use smaller local shops with higher prices than large supermarkets. The stress of living in poor or crowded conditions, constantly struggling to make ends meet, raises chances of stress-related illnesses such as cardiovascular disorders, hypertension and mental illness. Poorer housing areas often have inadequate recreation areas.

Who is to blame? – ideology and inequality

Although we know that opportunity is unequally and unfairly distributed, myths about poverty and inequality are perpetuated. They include ideas that the poor should try harder to escape their deprivations, that they are ignorant and lazy or, as discussed earlier, that they do little to fight the culture of poverty.

A key to the persistence of inequality is ideology. The most marked examples of how this works are offered by rigid systems of inequality which are supported by religious beliefs – the Hindu caste system offers an example. Such beliefs suggest that hierarchy is immutable and we can do nothing to change things in this life, nor should we since it is divinely ordained.

Similarly, quasi-religious justifications for extremes of inequality are commonly offered in the West. Inequality is seen as part of a natural order which is necessary to inspire people to succeed and thus should not be interfered with. Political leaders such as Margaret Thatcher and Ronald Reagan came to power offering ideological statements which supported existing inequalities. They argued that equality meant sameness and removing inequality would remove the differences between us, the things that made life exciting. Perhaps this justified not striving to remove inequality throughout the era of individualism and materialism in the 1980s.

However, just because people are different, it does not mean that we have to treat them unequally. What matters is that people are given equal opportunity to remedy cumulative disadvantages. We discuss how that might be accomplished in later chapters.

Power to change

A central problem is that the poor are rarely in a position to do anything about their own plight. They might appear to have as many political rights as everyone else but, in the same way that there is a cumulative culture of poverty, so too there is **cumulative political deprivation**. As discussed in Chapter 2, we need access to resources in order to achieve political ends and engage in sustained organised pressure.

By definition the poor lack such resources. For example, they lack the money, the valued skills and the influence with which to bargain in their own interests. If they had such resources, they would not be poor in the first place. Organising a political demonstration or a pressure group could prove impossible. The poor may not have much in common other than their poverty, and they may include categories of people who are in poverty for many different reasons: the unemployed, the old, the sick, the disabled, the homeless, the mentally ill, low-paid workers, immigrants, single-parent families and so on. People in poverty are very often reluctant or unable to organise in the first place. Low-paid female workers offer a case in point: they are a heterogeneous grouping, lacking similar interests other than their poverty.

Typical lobbying or pressure group operations involve regular interaction with influential politicians and state officials. The poor are less able to sustain this, and they possess neither the education nor the network of contacts to facilitate this. Instead, they rely on others to organise lobbying and pressure group activities on their behalf, apart from occasional direct action such as a rent strike. Once again this has been used to argue that the poor do not do enough to help themselves, that they could escape the poverty trap if they tried hard enough. The one element of truth in this is the irony that the calculated degradation of state welfare provision requires a kind of acceptance of the culture of poverty to succeed. Welfare and social security benefits are all part of the way of life of the poor. Survival in poverty depends upon gaining familiarity and expertise with welfare principles.

Conclusion

We have shown in this chapter that social inequality and the lack of social opportunity have a common-sense reality in society in so far as humans have priorities about certain resources. They differ in their access to these resources, and they distinguish between one another in terms of these resources. All of this has consequences for other opportunities in life.

On a subjective level it is of no use telling senior citizens in a city in an advanced industrial society that they are better off than peasants in rural India if they feel relatively deprived of something which they regard as essential to living. Similarly, even in subsistence terms, what may be regarded as a minimum acceptable level for living in rural India might not be tolerated in Western Europe. Poverty is relative to a community. Even objective measures of inequality have to take into account the general expectations of living standards in a particular community.

The study of social inequality is important for health professionals since health is dependent upon life chances. We are liable to suffer from certain illnesses or diseases according to the social category to which we belong. We cannot explain why some people are healthier than others by reference to physical, anatomical or physiological factors alone, but we do know that class, gender and ethnic group have a significant bearing on health. In the next three chapters we look at the sociological explanations for variations in life and health chances between these social categories.

Further reading

Bywaters, P. and McLeod, E. (1996) *Working for Equality in Health*, London: Routledge.
Practical considerations for action on inequality and health.

Sen, A. (1992) *Inequality Re-examined*, Oxford: Clarendon Press.
A comprehensive comparative discussion of inequality by an international economist.

Wilkinson, R.G. (1996) *Unhealthy Societies: The Afflictions of Inequality*, London: Routledge.
A readable comparative discussion of the connections between health and inequality.

Chapter 8 Inherited Health

The evidence connecting social class to health outcomes is overwhelming. The lower one moves down the class hierarchy, the higher the incidence of disease and relative mortality. This suggests that something in the attitudes, knowledge and behaviour of the social classes has a direct consequence on their access to and use of health and social care resources. Alternatively, there may be something in how the social classes interact with health and care workers to account for such differentials. We look first at the various theoretical perspectives on class, which aids understanding systematic variations in social class and health.

Theories of class inequality

A range of sociological theories explain how social inequality based on class occurs. Until the eighteenth century people talked of **rank** when distinguishing between social groups hierarchically. The term 'social class' emerged during the industrial revolution.

Marx's (1864) views have had a far-reaching influence on our understanding of class inequality. He saw class as hinging on whether or not people own the means of production. The main social classes have opposing sets of interests. The **bourgeoisie** (owners) want to make profits, and the **proletariat** (non-owners) want decent standards of living. The struggle between these two main classes is seen as the motor which drives historical development and social change. Capitalist society, dominated by the bourgeoisie, is the latest form of society to emerge from the struggle between two major social groups to achieve their interests. However, Marx pointed out that there were inherent contradictions within capitalism, not least from the material and social costs of constantly trying to lower the price of labour. He predicted that capitalists would need to create ever-larger monopolies in the attempt to secure profits, driving smaller entrepreneurs out of business. These larger monopolies could force down the price and value of labour. As a consequence working people would not be able to stay healthy enough to work or to sustain levels of education which would provide them with the skills needed to service a modern technology.

Marx also highlighted the importance of ideological processes in maintaining the acceptance by the subordinate class of their position. Such processes keep them ignorant about the possibility of achieving their own interests or even convince them that social inequality is somehow natural. Marx saw religion as the social institution most responsible for accomplishing this acceptance of a natural order. Even contemporary views of sickness as part of a natural order discourage people from taking real control of and responsibility for their own health. Marx went on to argue that eventually, as the proletariat becomes even poorer, and with the help of political groups which could raise their consciousness, they would have to overthrow the bourgeoisie in order to survive. He hoped that this would eventually lead to the creation of a **classless society** with no private ownership of the means of production.

Weber (1925) broadened the understanding of social class inequality. He saw **life chances** as the main criterion of class membership, determined by the skills and resources which can be offered in return for goods and services. Thus ownership of property will still influence one's life chances, since property can be exchanged for valued goods and services. However, Weber pointed out that **property varies in quantity and type**. Not all property owners possess equally marketable property and, as a result, their life chances differ. Similarly, those who do not own property differ in the kind of labour they can offer in the market. Thus the owner of a large factory is in a superior class position to a small shopkeeper, and a doctor is in a superior class position to a road sweeper, since the income returned for the goods and services they offer varies greatly. For this reason, as the capitalist economy grew more complex, it no longer made sense to talk of only two main classes. Many more classes could emerge, depending on the different types of property available and the different range of skills which people had to offer.

The importance of life chances in people gaining access to resources which help maintain their health is evident. Being able to afford the time and the cost for a holiday offers an illustration.

Exercise

Conduct an analysis of your own life chances.

What goods, services and lifestyles do you aspire to?

What are your chances of achieving them?

What property or skills do you possess that can be traded for those opportunities which you value?

Compare your own life chances with those of colleagues, clients or friends. Do they take some opportunities for granted which you would like to have?

Weber also pointed out that Marx's stress on the economic causes of inequality leads to a neglect of other influences, such as **social prestige** and **political power**. For Weber it was not enough to see social change and the development of capitalism as arising solely from economic class struggle. As we discussed in Chapter 2, prestige and power give differential access to valued resources and therefore shape social inequalities.

Moreover, Weber did not see religious ideas as excusing the iniquities of capitalism. Instead, he argued that the rise of the Protestant religion in particular had a fundamental influence on why and how capitalism developed. The moral force of hard work for the sake of God and not spending the profits of labour on selfish interests accounts for the rapid growth of modern capitalism. As we indicate in Chapter 6 the strength of such a religious ethic also explains the moral duty which is widely felt about working hard even today. Thus people see hard work as a healthy thing to do since it is morally advocated. This may be why they work harder than they should for the good of their own health.

Functionalist theorists, such as Davis and Moore (1967), do not see class inequality as a historical 'accident'. They have argued that social inequality is a natural part of the social order. Inequality is seen as providing a reward structure which motivates people to work hard and to take on the responsible tasks needed for the survival of a society. Functionalists argue that the stratification system works as a series of grades united through a **consensus on values**; that is, people in society agree on those values and with the system of status and prestige whereby people receive greater rewards for their social contribution. Functionalists reason that status rather than class is the most important social grouping, and that status arises out of consensus rather than conflict. This is diametrically opposed to the conflict view of society taken by Marx. For functionalists, conflict does not exist between the strata as such but between the individuals competing to move between the strata. In this view social stratification contributes to maintaining a consensus about values in a society and to integrating individuals within a social system. Despite being criticised this view persists and represents a popularly held view about the reasons for the existence of class inequality.

Contemporary views on class and health

Different theories of class inequality have different implications for health. All the theories can be used to explain the positive correlation between social class and illness. Marxist or conflict theories do this in terms of the economics of class – some groups are more privileged than others. Weberian views detail this by underlining the importance of skills and knowledge improving an individual's market position, status, power and therefore life chances. Functionalists might argue that unequal access to health resources is part of a natural social order, so society should get healthier as the ill disappear in a process of natural selection.

The functionalist view fits a politically conservative ideology and appears to justify existing class divisions. It becomes less feasible to argue for the power of inequality to motivate where continuing and cumulative advantages and disadvantages exist. Functionalists exaggerate the openness of the class system. It is not possible for everyone to attain rewards that remain scarce. In contrast, conflict theorists suggests that the view that openness exists represents **false consciousness** in that it supports an ideological illusion that anyone can make it to the top of the hierarchy if they strive hard enough.

Indeed, contemporary evidence suggests other flaws in the functionalist perspective. The World Bank has argued that reducing the extremes of inequality is an important determinant of growth in developing countries. The more an economy can integrate all its people into national development, the greater their skills, the larger their incomes and the more rapid the economic growth for that society. Carrying a large proportion of the community as poor and unskilled appears to be a social and economic burden that holds an economy back. South East Asia, the region of highest economic growth in the world, is one of the least unequal regions.

The validity of the conflict perspective might have been tested in the communist regimes of the former Soviet Union, Eastern Europe and China. In East European socialist societies, however, while ownership of goods did not distinguish greatly between people, there were class distinctions between a 'productive' class and a 'redistributor' class. The latter included technocrats, bureaucrats and intelligentsia who made the decisions about what counted as legitimate expropriation and redistribution of surplus goods. Similarly, in the People's Republic of China between 1950 and the mid-1980s status was more important than money. It could buy more space, better working conditions, better food and deference which could, in turn, allow those who had status access to further benefits. Consequently, it is argued, social class did not disappear after the revolutions in either of these societies.

Social, economic and political change has been so great that it is difficult to assess the appropriateness of different theories. Modern societies are pluralist in that they are more multicultural and we all receive a variety of different ideas from the breadth of mass communication sources now available. One theoretical view is that the Marxist approach has been undermined by the growth of a **post-capitalist** society in which the extremes of conflict have been moderated by institutionalised bargaining procedures and the provision of state welfare. This view also holds that mobility between the social classes is high and, since there are many new and different occupations, classes are less distinct and less opposed to each other.

An opposite view is that capitalism has not fundamentally altered and, if anything, indicators of inequality point to an increasing crisis in the system which may be concealed only for so long. People's expectations of improved living standards and working conditions must be increasingly frustrated so that the **crisis of capitalism** will worsen and radical forms of dissent will increase. However, both perspectives point out how **ideology** is vital in determining how or whether the state will continue to operate with legitimacy in the face of persistent social inequalities.

Current theoretical views contain elements of the above theories and require understanding class inequality in terms of four major influences:

1. **Wealth.** Ownership or non-ownership of productive wealth remains the most important determinant of life chances since it is a significant determinant of access to scarce goods and services. As we discuss in Chapter 7, wealth permits lifestyles which secure better health resources.

2. **The labour market.** The developed division of labour in complex societies means that life chances are significantly affected by the market for abilities, skills, talent, education or training. Knowledge and expertise command resources if there is demand for them. It cannot be assumed that the market for such skills is free or open. Government, professional association or trade union activities can control the supply of skills, thereby raising their price. The extent of the division of labour does complicate the class structure: the more varied the skills and expertise available or demanded, the greater the range of class positions.

Key questions

What has happened to the ability of professions allied to medicine to command a price for their skills in the health labour market?

What effects have these developments had on the price for or value of doctors' skills?

Think about how nurses' class positions might alter as they are educated to higher standards and take on more clinical responsibilities. As new grades of assistant health care workers are introduced the position of nurses may improve. Care assistants, too, are gaining more formal qualifications. The emerging role of nurse practitioner alters the position of junior doctors in the labour market. Similarly, other medically related professionals, such as radiographers, are being educated to higher levels, and their skills become more differentiated as new radiographic techniques are introduced.

3. **The workplace.** The developing and changing division of labour also brings more complexity to workplace activity. The

nature of work tasks, the people you relate to in work and the power or authority you acquire from work tasks all exert crucial influences on the way you feel about yourself or perceive the world, both on and off the job. Again the variations in these relationships create a complexity in the social stratification hierarchy. Thus some people with a very low level of training can hold a great deal of power to influence the lives of others.

Exercise

Using the means for conducting a political analysis we introduced in Chapter 2, analyse the power of:

● a traffic warden;

● the clerk who deals with your banking, insurance, income tax or medical records and who has access to personal records held about you on computer databases;

● the doctor's receptionist.

Similarly, people's cultural predispositions and therefore their attitudes and behaviour can be influenced by workplace relations in a way which bears no link to their economic position. In the workplace you may come across new practices which introduce you to ideas you would never have experienced in your home community or locale.

Exercise

Do you remember learning of people's habits, practices, tastes and dispositions in the workplace which you had never come across before?

---

4. **Cultural heterogeneity**. Finally, the wide variety of modern leisure activities provides extra grounds for differentiating between people and also bringing together groups who may

be divided in other, more traditional settings. Sporting activities, foreign travel, multimedia activities and dining out are all activities which allow people to cross traditional boundaries of class, status and power.

Exercise

Think about your own leisure activities. What sort of people have you met and interacted with... on holiday; at the gym; in your amateur dramatics association; in a club... and so on? Are these people with whom you might not normally associate?

Consequences of social inequality for health

One of the major contributions that sociology has made to the explanation of health and illness is to aid understanding of the social factors lying behind patterns of disease and illness. When we introduced the major theoretical perspectives in Chapter 1, we pointed out how theories fell into two main categories: structural perspectives with macro-sociological concerns and processual perspectives with micro-sociological concerns.

The knowledge which supports structural theories tends to be based on quantitative data, while processual or interactionist approaches seek more qualitative data. Put simply, the difference between these perspectives is that, on the one hand, 'structure imposes constraints on how humans interact' and, on the other, 'repeated interaction create structures'. Thus the two are really interconnected, as Giddens' structuration theory implies. Full sociological explanation requires putting the two approaches together.

Structural constraints on health

Structural approaches look for patterns in human groups or systematic social behaviour. They have to employ broad principles of categorisation which may overwhelm individual behaviour, but they are essential to pinpoint trends. It is in this connection that **social epidemiology** has made contributions. Epidemiology is the study of the quantifiable features of groups of people which may explain prevalences of morbidity and mortality for those groups. Indicators such as employment rates, levels of educational attainment, family size, gender, age, ethnicity and social class are correlated with morbidity (illness) and mortality (death) rates. It is from such work that the consistent relationship between social class and health has been demonstrated (Kaplan *et al*. 1993).

There has been much argument over the validity and reliability of such indicators. As we discuss in Chapter 7, some see social class, as measured by occupational scales, as a rather crude indicator of social inequality. Much the same could be said for indicators of health. The most common measure is **self-reported health status**, which entails asking people how they feel and how they respond to the performance of selected routine, mundane tasks. Epidemiology largely falls back on a medical model and employs indicators of mortality and morbidity. The assumption is that those not ill or dying must be (relatively) healthy. Most public health policy is devised in light of these broad measures (Blane *et al*. 1996).

Evidence of inequalities in treatment provision can be seen in the way in which some diseases are treated as being of more concern than others and tackled in a narrow way. For example, cardiovascular complaints disproportionately affect the working class, but very little effort is put into preventive measures which confront their lifestyle (diet, work conditions, leisure habits and so on). There are many regional variations in epidemiology which suggest localised and community-related problems which could be collectively confronted. Instead, major effort goes into heart transplants and coronary bypass surgery, which can only ever deal with the problems of a minority, which is funded by the existence of enough high-paying customers and which produces prestige and an elite status within the medical profession.

Healthy social processes

Evidently, some groups of people acquire access to facilities and resources to maintain their health while others do not. Life chances are linked to health chances, but does 'chance' mean the **opportunity** to engage in particular health-related behaviours?

Exercise

What do you do to stay healthy?

What resources do you employ to do that?

What groups of people lack access to these valued health and care resources?

Take one group or individual with which you have some familiarity and ask:

● why can't they gain access to such resources?

● what are their barriers to equal access to health?

By now you should have the means for conducting a fairly comprehensive analysis of these sorts of issue. Think about, for example, knowledge, information, ideology, cultural norms and habituated behaviour, and how they play a part in the way in which people take advantage of their chances. Include processes such as potential role conflicts, conflicting wants and needs, and conflicting interests and how they might inhibit access to health.

In most societies the groups who lack such resources are the poor, the homeless, the unemployed and those lowest down the social class hierarchy. These are often the same people.

We introduced the idea of equality of opportunity for education in Chapter 5. It was used to indicate the view that, despite marked differences in social backgrounds, all children should begin with the same educational chances. How does this apply to **equality of access to health**? Blaxter (1996) and Whitehead and Dahlgren (1991) use the concept of equity to explore attempts to redistribute health resources more fairly. Equity means ensuring a form of positive discrimination: getting health resources to those who need it most but who are less able to use their own resources to seek health. The British National Health Service could not do this given its primary concern with treating illness.

Part of the problem relates to the difference between the structure of social inequality and how people experience it. How do you know whether you are not getting equal access to health facilities and resources? Few ordinary patients are aware of the background constraints on the work of their health carers. How much time can be allowed for the patient? What are the financial implications of different treatments to the doctor, the hospital and the patient? The patient has knowledge of their own costs but not those of the health care service. Some practitioners take decisions not to tell patients about expensive treatment if they assume them to be unable to afford it.

Those who are able to take advantage of health facilities and amenities treat it as part of their expected normal practices. Going to the gym, taking a weekend break, a skiing holiday, a beach holiday, are things that some people take for granted. Choosing to pay for treatment from alternative therapists or complementary medicine may not even be contemplated by other people. Drinking to excess, eating the wrong sorts of food, fighting in a bar or at a sports event, and smoking cigarettes are all part of routine cultural activity for some groups.

The kinds of health hazard one is exposed to at work varies between the social classes. The risks in work such as heavy industry, building or mining are part of the job while the risks from **sick building syndrome** may be much more subtle. Even apparently protected working environments such as modern offices or modern hospitals can have damaging forms of fluorescent lighting, poor ventilation and excessive formaldehyde in furnishing materials, to say nothing of work technologies which may induce repetitive strain injuries. It is not that the upper and middle classes suffer no health risks, but they will be categorised differently.

Exercise

Make observations of risky health behaviour, health-inducing and illness-inducing practices you come across over the next few days or which you read about in the newspapers.

Be imaginative and open to novel sources of risk.

Consider how risks link to specific social class, occupation, gender, ethnic or age groupings.

Here are some we have come across:

- **Double-dipping corn chips at parties** – that is, placing the chip in the dip, biting off the dipped bit and then redipping into the communal dip, even though the chip has touched the lips.

- **Helping yourself to the free peanuts on the bar** – a study in one bar showed traces of twelve different types of urine on the communal peanuts. Who does not wash their hands after visiting the toilet?

- **Sharing a cigarette** – not just sharing a packet but passing a cigarette from the mouth of one person to another.

- **Unsterilised stethoscopes** – how often do health care practitioners sterilise their instruments? Certainly not between every patient, but between how many patients? One study found traces of *Staphylococcus aureus* on one in every five stethoscopes. How many practitioners wash their hands properly between hands-on care of a patient? More think they do than actually do.

An appreciation of a person's economic and cultural background and domestic circumstances is essential if holistic health care is to be given. Consideration of such influences affects treatment, prognosis and conditions of discharge from care. Health education or advice is wasted if it does not match the background circumstances of the client. Given their previous experience of dealing with state officials, some groups resent and resist health and social care professionals as representatives of social control agencies. Professionals may be seen as interfering or simply not able to understand the problems faced by clients who have fundamentally different socio-economic and cultural experiences.

Conclusion: How fixed is social inequality?

The consequences of structured social inequalities depend on how far a specific system of social inequality lasts over time. Can unfairness and inequality of opportunity be removed if the fundamental bases of inequality change? In part, this depends on whether or not...

1. **...criteria for ranking or evaluating people are systematically transmitted from one generation to the next.** Those born into certain groups will be socialised into expecting different life experiences and life chances from those born into other

groups. Such expectations are passed on through education, work and home situations, legislation and cultural habits.

2. **...the resources which underpin criteria for social classification continue to be important and valued**. The importance to society of the skills and resources on which criteria for evaluating differences are based will change if there is a revolution or resources suddenly become less scarce. Thus if everyone received the same income, income would no longer serve as an adequate criterion on which to differentiate between people. A sense of resource scarcity is the key to differentiation. Thus health has been a key commodity in the West for about two hundred years. Only a minority could afford it until the early twentieth century. It became so vital to the supply of human resources in the advanced industrial nations that they devised schemes for ensuring the health of the bulk of the population, providing some state welfare and health services. Ironically, this became vital in the preparations for the First World War, keeping working men fit enough to fight. It was for this reason that doctors commanded a high price. What if health became less valued? Or so scarce and valued that the health policy of the Ik tribe mentioned in Chapter 1 became generally applied. Not spending resources on the aged or infirm conserves the scarce resources needed to keep the young alive.

3. **...how far social mobility, or movement between social groups can take place**. How easy is it for workers to become managers? Are we rigidly set into castes from which we cannot escape? Clearly, if social mobility were frequent – if individuals were able to move rapidly from one class to another – the whole basis of the classification system would be eroded. If we have all been impoverished at some time in our lives, we may have more sympathy for those currently in poverty. On the other hand, if we have escaped poverty, we may find it hard to understand why others cannot do the same.

As we said earlier, being different does not have to mean being unequal. Gender remains a source of social differentiation that is unlikely to change. In Chapter 9 we consider why gender is productive of such durable inequalities and the consequences of this for health care.

Further reading

The following articles take these issues further:

Jenkins, R. (1991) 'Disability and social stratification', *British Journal of Sociology*, **42**: 557–80.

Oakley, A. and Rajan, L. (1991) 'Social class and social support – the same or different?', *Sociology*, **25**: 31–59.

Vagero, D. (1991) 'Inequality in health – some theoretical and empirical problems', *Social Science and Medicine*, **32**: 367–71.

White, K. (1991) 'The sociology of health and illness', *Current Sociology*, **39**: 1–115.

Chapter 9 Natural Carers: Sex and Gender

Differences in the health chances of men and women are lifelong. Gender relations are commonly seen as being determined by women's biological potential for childbearing, but we must recognise how women's health is governed more by social than by biological differences.

In most Western industrial societies, women have gained legal equality with men. Only a few decades ago women could not expect to be able to vote, find similar employment or be given equal access to education. However, women are still paid consistently less than men, they are more likely to live in poverty, especially in later life, and they carry the greater burden of housework and domestic care responsibilities – all of which have health consequences.

Gender imagery

Any social role, including that of being a woman or a man, is built from expectations reflecting the attitudes, norms and values of the larger society. We gain insights into these expectations if we look at the vocabulary and labels which we use to depict men and women as different. The use of such labels supports social practices which separate men and women by reinforcing stereotypes.

Exercise

List the traits or characteristics which you would associate with a 'female' image. Then list their equivalent (and opposite?) 'male' traits.   *cont'd*

144

> How would you characterise yourself in relation to any of the traits you have listed?
>
> How far do you think you fit your stereotyped image for your own sex? How well do you think this fits with your image of being a health carer?
>
> If you have designated yourself as having displayed any 'opposite sex' traits, recall any example of recent activities in which you see yourself as having expressed these. How favourable or un-favourable were the reactions of other people to your doing so?

This exercise produces vocabulary such as 'strong', 'thought-ful', 'intelligent', 'sensitive', 'emotional' and so on. Make your list as long as possible and then compare some of your imagery with that of a friend or partner or colleague.

Words that are exclusively applied to men and women provide the basis for **sexism** – stereotypical attitudes and expectations which differentiate sharply between males and females, and which restrict their behaviour.

Such fundamental social arrangements are often displayed and affirmed in ceremonial and ritualised ways. As we outlined in Chapter 3, ways have to be found in which to exhibit social roles and their relationship to each other. When gender is displayed it indicates sexual identity and relationships between the sexes. As with many role performances, gender displays represent ideal rather than real relationships.

To illustrate, mass communications succeed by constructing simple but effective messages using conventions to portray idealised relationships. Kuhn (1985) has pointed out how their subtle conventions of visual imagery carry direct messages about types of people and ways of behaving that impose stringent social constraints, especially in the area of sexual identity. Traditionally, as gender images lend themselves to simple dichotomies, the presentation of sexual identity as uncompromising opposites has been an easy message to convey.

Modern mass media have also contributed to contemporary aesthetics by constructing culturally acceptable views of the human body. These images play an important part in establishing what counts as fashionable, beautiful or healthy. Economic and technological developments have increased pressures for novelty in the media business. This means that such images about bodies and gender may be allowed to change more rapidly.

In both the construction and interpretation of images, the conventions which help us to make sense of an image are part of the underlying **grammar of visual imagery**. Goffman (1979) suggested the following as a few of the conventions which are used to indicate and interpret gender identity and relations:

- the ranking of **functions**: the gender division of labour; who does what work;
- **hierarchy**, represented by relative body size;
- **subordination**, indicated through body posture;
- **touch** and the use of hands: females as gently touching; men as firmly grasping;
- **objectification**: the implication that what is being represented can be treated as an object;
- **fragmentation**: when the body is not seen as a whole but as a summation of body parts, thereby further enhancing objectification.

Exercise

Collect some visual materials – advertisements from women's or men's magazines, newspaper colour supplements, television advertisements, pictures from medical or health journals.
Examine them according to Goffman's criteria.

Studying such visual materials highlights representations of women and men in terms of their relative power, as authoritative or responsible figures in different contexts. The contrast between how men and women are represented in work, domestic and leisure settings is noteworthy. Are women treated more as 'objects'?

Theories of gender differences

Sociological analyses of gender relations have drawn on a range of theoretical approaches. Social stratification theorists such as John Goldthorpe (1983) argue that patterns of social inequality should be understood through analysing the family as a unit. The social and economic position of a family is usually determined by that of the breadwinner. Since breadwinners are mostly male, the role of women in the analysis of inequality becomes marginalised. This view has been criticised on the basis that there are important gender inequalities in the distribution of resources and power within the family. Many households are neither family units, nor headed by males. Women's contribution to families in terms of their income, employment and other aspects of their work is distinctive and needs to be addressed.

A **liberal feminist** approach details the obstacles that have to be overcome by women as they gain access to a range of resources from health care to employment. If these obstacles, such as the timing of surgery opening hours or lack of child care support, were removed, a more equal relationship between the sexes could be built.

Marxist feminists put forward a wider explanation for gender inequalities. They link the exploitation of women as unpaid workers to the needs of the capitalist system to reproduce itself. Housewives produce children and provide forms of unpaid personal care within the household. This lowers the costs to the economic system of maintaining the workforce as well as holding down the market price of women's work outside the family and reducing their job security.

Radical feminists argue that all social institutions, including the family, education, politics and the media, alongside the economic system, are linked in generating gender-based inequalities in power. This makes it systematically possible for men's interests to dominate those of women. Such a system of gender dominance is called **patriarchy**. Evidence of patriarchy includes male violence and harassment towards women, heterosexual practices in which women's interests are not addressed and women's work generally being controlled by men.

Dual systems theorists argue that gender relations are structured by a combination of patriarchy and capitalism. The operations of the capitalist system limit the resources available to women to improve their position in the home, while patriarchy ensures their continued exclusion from better-paid, more secure jobs in the wider labour market.

Postmodernists point out the dangers of overstating the similarities between women and therefore overlooking important social differences in the forms of gender relations. For example, it could be argued that relationships between men and women are structured very differently within different race, class and historical contexts.

Women and work

Male traits are more typically associated with the world of formal work. Women's activities may not be called work, but they support the ability of men to function in the world of work. This allocates women a secondary role dependent on men's primary roles. Such variations in the distribution of power shape men's and women's access to and control over care-related activities and resources. This calls into question the degree to which women's roles as unpaid carers are 'natural'.

Resources are made available to most people through employment. Examining gender inequalities in employment can reveal the dynamics which link public and private pressures on women's caring. Women, on average, earn less than men since they tend to be employed part time and in poorly paid occupations and industries.

Women's family commitments affect their career patterns (Poland 1992). They are more likely to take a career break when they are having children. Many women returners to work are unable to take jobs using the same skills at the same level of pay that they had before leaving. Women also find that they need to work part time to accommodate child care and other domestic commitments. These jobs are less likely to be as skilled, and neither are they likely to be supported by employment protection, benefits or pensions.

One consequence of women's different relationship with employment is the **vertical segregation** of women within the labour market. They are most likely to be found in high numbers in the lower grades of occupations and hardly to be found at all at the highest grades. The difficulty women have in securing promotion at the highest levels is popularly known as the **glass ceiling** phenomenon – seeing the 'upper floors' but not being able to get there (Poland *et al.* 1996). A second consequence is the **horizontal segregation** of women into different occupations from men. Women are most likely to be found in professions relating to health and welfare, and least likely to be found in professions related to management or technology. They are also especially likely to be found in personal service occupations and in clerical work. They are least likely to be found in heavy industrial work, transport or communications.

Women are not necessarily less skilled or less well educated than men, but their circumstances constrain them to take less well-paid jobs. As we indicated in Chapter 6 global economic trends are encouraging more flexible jobs linked with part-time work and traditionally female-predominant occupations, such as clerical and care work. As long-term health care moves out of hospitals, and many community care tasks become the responsibility of contracted care agencies, there will be higher numbers of insecure, hourly-paid personal care jobs, supervised by health professionals and care managers.

Key questions

In what ways may women's employed work affect their health chances?

Women's work has been linked to fatigue and burn-out as a result of work with long and irregular hours, anxiety and depression caused by lack of power over their work and low esteem, giving their own health and diet a lower priority than that of their family and reduced time for leisure or exercise.

Feminists have played an important part in highlighting aspects of inequality within gender relations and encouraging political and economic responses to them. Equity in pay and employment is now a widely accepted policy principle. Violence against women is also now taken seriously as a social problem to be officially addressed rather than as a domestic issue. The difficulties of finding practical solutions to gender inequality show how gender relations are embedded in wider patterns of social interaction.

Exercise

Find some articles featuring women's occupations drawn from:

● a tabloid newspaper;

● a trades union publication;

● a women's glossy magazine;

● a health-promotion publication.

What theoretical approach is represented by the perspective taken by the writer of each article?

What theoretical perspectives might you use to explain the approaches taken by each type of publication?

Women as health carers

Feminist perspectives have encouraged increasing agreement that the subordination of women is grounded in a division of labour which is linked to, but not caused by, the different reproductive roles of men and women. Being a wife, a mother and a hetero-sexual are relational roles to men. Such a division of labour is institutionalised in the family and reflected in the wider society.

Although women's roles are so closely linked to the reproduction of society itself, feminists argue that there are reasons why these roles do not confer economic or political power to control the conditions of that reproduction. Women are essential providers of everyday health, yet they are viewed as troublesome if not confined to particular roles. Feminists argue that this confinement of women to specific roles in the reproduction of society is achieved by over-identifying them with functions of biological reproduction. Asserting the 'naturalness' of such roles obscures their social value and allows the stigma of 'unnatural' to be applied to women moving outside such roles.

Thus, even in professional health care, the glass ceiling operates. While the vast majority of workers in the health care system are women, they are concentrated at the bottom of the medical occupational hierarchy. In the UK nearly 90 per cent of nurses, but only about 20 per cent of doctors, are women, with very few at the top of the medical profession. Men dominate the better-paid technical and organisationally responsible roles. In contrast, those jobs involving the most practical, day-to-day care of patients attract much less pay and status, and are occupied by women (Riska and Wegar 1993).

Exercise

Note any examples of how gender relations influence partnerships in health work which you have come across.

Are there noticeable gender differences in authority, status, working conditions, pay, talk and body language?

This pattern of relationships has a long history linked to the rise of the modern medical profession, displacing a tradition of predominantly female lay healers, from herbalists to midwives. As specialist occupations developed throughout modern society women were increasingly excluded from medical care. This even happened in midwifery, in which women were banned from using the forceps invented by male barber-surgeons. Women were relegated to the subordinate role of helpers as the male medical profession became increasingly technologically oriented and economically powerful.

Medicalising women

It has been further argued that women's bodies have been used as sites for a variety of social and medical sanctions. Men dominate the medical profession, which, in turn, dominates the health care system. Much attention has been given to the need to reassert female self-confidence by **demedicalising** such natural female functions as menstruation, conception, pregnancy and childbearing. Such challenges centre on definitions of health and the treatment of illness.

At the end of the twentieth century women in Western countries are living on average seven years longer than men. However, they are found to report higher occurrences of illness and to be major consumers of health care. They suffer fewer infectious or degenerative diseases than men but more psychological and longer-term chronic illnesses.

Research has suggested that domestic responsibilities give women more opportunities to demonstrate sick role behaviour. However, feminists have argued that these morbidity rates are not simply an artefact of illness behaviour. The physical symptoms reported, rates of long-term illness and rates of primary care consultation on stress are linked to women's class and race. This may indicate that their health chances follow from aspects of their work and family responsibilities (Graham 1993).

Women are accorded responsibility for informal care. When resources for families are in short supply women often protect family members by self-deprivation. However, this cannot work when the problems stem from a socio-economic context which is beyond their control, as with trends in employment or transport. The wider society may make women, as mothers, individually responsible for health tasks such as breast-feeding and attendance at antenatal and child clinics. Yet patterns of employment and transport make the performance of these tasks problematic. In such cases problems stemming from wider social responsibilities for health are likely to be attributed to 'poor mothering'.

Marked class, age and gender differences are seen in access rates for medical services. These are most significant for women in the less-skilled and unskilled working classes who are least likely to be referred for specialist services by family practitioners. Older, lower-class women are the group least likely to be referred.

It is often suggested, especially by policy-makers, that working-class women may have 'less healthy' health beliefs or lifestyle choices, which would explain such illness and referral rates. However, structural factors such as employment and resources, rather than lifestyle factors such as diet and exercise, are most closely implicated. It appears to be skill in using health provision rather than their health beliefs which has the greatest effect on their access to services. Although women are the biggest users of health care facilities, they do so less on their own behalf than as child carers and supporters of other people's health. Medicine therefore affects women to a much greater extent than it does men. Feminists have emphasised the need for women to share skills and support in negotiating with health services. The women's movement in the USA has encouraged the spread of direct, collective health action by women.

Women may prefer to avoid contact with medical professionals if they are only offered medical advice or interventions in place of other kinds of support. If the weight of advice emphasises individual responsibility, this may be further isolating. Diverse forms of support may be needed as not everyone receives the same degree of support from their families.

Parallel patterns of gender subordination may be seen in women's access to and roles in sport – a health-associated leisure activity – and in the health risks of new technologies. Accepting a notion of gender relations means recognising that attempts to address women's health entails a focus on the wider cultural and social context of women's health.

Access to resources supporting health

The health care choices of poorer women are especially constrained. Graham (1993) has emphasised how the task of providing household care on a limited budget brings additional responsibilities without power. The ability to survive may mean drawing on whatever routines and non-financial resources women have access to, such as time out to talk with friends, have a cup of coffee, take a bath or pray. Few of these are readily recognisable as health resources. Activities such as smoking or dependence on tranquillisers may be seen as unhealthy in the long run but may offer necessary support in the short term.

Taking on care-giving responsibilities can restrict women's access to other opportunities which might support their self-care and thereby their health chances. These might include working overtime, taking opportunities for retraining or extra qualifications, attending social functions which give access to networks, jobs with better pensions and leisure activities.

Key questions

Present trends in health care are increasingly shifting the longer-term health care of older, physically disabled and other dependent groups away from hospitals and formal health settings and into the community. The bulk of such care is likely to be undertaken by women in domestic settings.

cont'd

What social factors are likely to affect the provision of resources to support such work?

What are likely to be the needs of unpaid carers undertaking such work?

Studies of care-giving have highlighted the degree to which carers may be called on to balance competing commitments. However, because work in the home is less visible, its demands on carers are hidden from the wider society. These may be further hidden because stress or inability to cope is often seen as a personal failure in performing care-giving roles.

Such 'failures' can also be consequential for the kinds of medical treatment which women receive. Studies of patterns of interaction between patients and health professionals have highlighted how patients may be categorised as good or bad according to the amount of 'trouble' they cause in health work settings. Women are seen as more troublesome because they are more likely to present with 'untreatable' emotional, psychiatric and chronic diseases. Assessments of their goodness as wives, employees and mothers will also be brought to bear in assessing their worthiness as health care participants, whether as patients or informal carers. Their categorisation as 'bad' is likely to lead to less information being given to them and to measures of control and sanctioning. Medicalisation of the domestic domain is increasingly taking place through health-related assessments of child care, domestic work, food preparation and family relationships.

Trends to medicalise social activities in the home may reinforce judgements about women's performance in particular roles. Feminists question whether wifehood and heterosexuality is always beneficial to women's mental and physical health. However, without other social changes, simply challenging the wifely role is not enough. If women are not guaranteed access to higher incomes through marriage, they are open to poverty. This seems to be reflected in higher levels of economic insecurity for women after divorce. This can only be counteracted if women's position in the labour market is strengthened to give them greater economic self-sufficiency.

Woman-friendly health care organisation and medical techniques

The problems many women experience in relation to food illustrates the tensions between women's performance as individual 'good carers' and their capacity to care for themselves and to obtain health support in doing so. Diverse calls on women's time heighten the attraction of providing meals through processed foods. It is ironic that popular images of feminine attractiveness highlight thinness, given women's greater involvement in food provision and preparation. Consequently, many women experience eating problems, ranging from dietary restrictions or obsessions to anorexia and bulimia.

Medical interventions to counteract eating problems, from weight gaining to weight loss diets or operations, carry their own health risks. Health action groups have pressed for organisational and social policy strategies to address such issues. These approaches may include putting pressure on schools to provide healthier food for children, diet participation groups at family practitioner clinics, carer support groups or joint campaigns with women health worker organisations.

Childbirth as health or illness

Different social groups can draw on different perspectives and resources to attempt to control life events. This is exemplified in the case of childbirth and whether medical or non-medical interventions and perspectives are likely to take precedence.

Key questions

Which of the following statements appears closest to the truth?

'Childbirth is a natural and life-enhancing event for women and their families.'

'Childbirth is a perilous, life-threatening event for women and their families.'

Childbirth may be treated as an illness because of the non-routine bodily changes and disruptions which women experience. Hospital as the most frequent place of birth, the involvement of health care professions and specialist medical technologies lead to treating childbirth as an illness. It may also be treated as a non-illness because of its 'normality' as a life event and in the everyday processes of family care work and its positive fulfilment of roles and gender expectations.

However, further reflection on the values, purposes, resources, language and skills used by different groups to frame such events points to how power dynamics influence their success in getting their views accepted. Take the problem of parental choice on where to give birth – at home or in hospital. Parents need a range of political resources to oppose whatever official maternity view is held at the time.

Childbirth is much more than a medical event. It is also a life event which can be seen as having a variety of effects on the life course of those involved, especially the woman, depending on the social context in which it takes place. As a rite of passage, childbirth can mark a woman's transition to particular rights as well as responsibilities as a mother. As a planned experience it can be timed and controlled to fit in with a woman's other commitments and priorities in a manageable way. As an unplanned event it can intervene in other plans or relationships in welcome or unwelcome ways. In the context of some social relationships this lack of choice can be experienced as coercion. In other contexts the associated changes in status and family relationships may make childbirth a source of power.

Longitudinal studies of women's experiences of pregnancy, childbirth and childrearing have stressed the changes that childbirth may bring to women's lives and relationships (Oakley 1979). Such accounts emphasise the need for women to share more realistic insights to reflect the mixture of experiences that maternity may bring. The use of women's own accounts can be contrasted with the treatment of obstetric information in medical textbooks, which may advance other views and preferences using technical language.

It is because of the social visibility of childbirth and its consequences for their life courses that some feminists argue that male control over women's reproduction is central to female subordination. Action taken to support greater control for women has included forming women's health groups, to share information about health and reproductive control, and setting up women's clinics, where women are able to consult other women about their health. There is increasing public support for women's right to choose whether they give birth at home with the help of a midwife, or in hospital. At present about 99 per cent of births in the UK take place in hospital rather than at home. The medical control of labour and delivery positions has also been challenged in relation to whether these are chosen to suit the medical staff or to assist the comfort and health of women giving birth.

Issues about empowerment can stem from the gendered nature of health occupations and their relative access to resources. These will affect how far midwives are able to support mothers in being empowered and also how far they can secure recognition for their skills and experience. Ann Oakley (1984) has compared the relative styles and responsibilities of midwives in a variety of European and North American countries. She contrasts their scope for exercising midwifery skills autonomously as opposed to performing supervised tasks within a more medical-dominated obstetric care context.

Exercise

Identify an aspect of midwifery practice you have recently observed or been involved with. Describe in what ways this may add to or detract from the resources available to:

- a woman to gain control of an aspect of her own pregnancy or childbirth;

- a midwife to gain control of an aspect of her work.

How far do your conclusions suggest that this aspect of practice is supportive of both women's concerns?

Impact of reproductive technologies

Feminists have attempted to modify the medical control of reproduction through the control of contraception, abortion and childbirth as well as other female 'troubles', such as the menopause. Giving birth, preventing birth or even having an abortion are not intrinsically medical concerns. Women are not necessarily, or even normally, ill in connection with giving birth, preventing birth or having an abortion. This is not to say that there are no illnesses which are related to these events. Attempts to demedicalise more aspects of reproduction are nonetheless vigorously resisted by gynaecological and obstetric medical specialities.

In contrast it is clear that if women are to maximise their health and the degree of control they have over their own working lives, they must be able to influence their reproductive lives in the wider sense. Such control only partly relates to their biological reproductive activities. Women have had to seek effective means of controlling their own fertility without risky side-effects and to make pregnancy and childbirth safer.

Developments in medical technology have generated a range of **reproductive technologies** which may affect both gender relations and the degree of control which women have over their own bodies. These developments have included hormonal interventions, intrauterine devices and techniques which may be used in contraception and also in conception, as well as genetic mapping.

Contraceptive developments have included hormonal pills, implants and barrier methods such as the diaphragm, and surgical interventions such as sterilisation. The birth control movement has proved a double-edged sword for women. The possibility for greater control over their own bodies which is offered to women may also be open to other agents, including the state. The weight of social pressures on women to have children or not undermines the notion that their choices here are only personal. Family ties, religion and national politics may all play a part in colouring such decisions. Contraceptive procedures which are less directly controllable by women themselves have often been more likely to be used with more socially vulnerable women such as black or working-class women. These include long-acting hormonal injections or implants. Developments in controlling reproduction cannot be simply seen as empowering for women.

There have also been criticisms of the role of medical staff in representing such technologies as unduly free of medical or social risks or discomforts. Fertility procedures such as in vitro fertilisation (IVF) and other procedures involving transferring or transplanting eggs or embryos can bring a number of hazards. Nearly all of them can adversely affect the health of the woman or the embryo or child. For IVF these include higher rates of prematurity, delivery by caesarean section, an increase in the chance of multiple births, and a higher percentage of babies with long-term health problems and major abnormalities, including neural tube and cardiac problems.

Most fertility procedures are expensive and access to them is therefore, in practice, restricted to those who can afford to pay. Furthermore, women who are not in stable, cohabiting relationships with men are not seen by medical gate-keepers as acceptable for motherhood by these means.

How far reproductive technologies can empower women will therefore depend on the contexts of power to which different groups of women in different societies have access. Powerful commercial interests dominate the provision of all reproductive technologies and, in the case of population control, are closely interlinked with governments and aid agencies. The initial enthusiasm of women's health activists has been modified as doubts have arisen about how **reproductive technologies may objectify women**. They point to the uses of such technologies in creating a more direct relationship between the wider society, medicine and the fetus and, by new means, further marginalising women's role.

The new genetics represented by the Human Genome Project seeks detailed links between specific genetic elements and human development, including congenital abnormalities, illnesses and even aspects of cognitive abilities and personality. These have opened up possibilities for genetic testing to aid modification of genetic materials or to guide decisions to abort fetuses with traits seen as problematic. The eugenic overtones in this development have been criticised as further objectifying women in reducing their role to that of embryo carrier.

Given the **gendered power differentials** in science, technology and the wider society, it is unlikely that women, who are most likely to be affected, will be those who will decide on what is or is not desirable in these new developments in reproduction. Such technologies may be justified as appropriate responses to infertility or unwanted reproduction without examining the wider causes of infertility or overfertility. Without a redistribution of power women are unlikely to be able to take a key role in reproductive decisions.

Key questions

Think about reproductive control in the relationships with which you have familiarity. What technologies are employed in enhancing

cont'd

---

or limiting fertility? What factors influence their employment – both directly, in terms of personal relationships, and indirectly, in terms of access, availability and information? How have these influences changed over time?

Reproductive technologies can strengthen male control over reproduction and reduce female control and visibility in this area. Given the view that women are their biology, and as that biology can be controlled through reproductive technologies, this can be successfully presented as improving choices for women. The 'need' to mother is one which is rarely socially questioned. A reduction to biology facilitates women's social disappearance while the rights of other interested parties are formulated. These include those of male partners and of the embryo as a social entity with an existence independent of the woman. In this way new reproductive technologies can as easily be seen as disempowering women as empowering them.

The medicalisation of sexual orientation

As well as being closely associated with biological reproduction **women's identities are also highly sexualised**. This is shown when women attempt to gain entry to settings or occupations from which they have been traditionally excluded. Their presence is often presented as being potentially sexually unsettling or distracting to male co-participants. An example of such disruption frequently raised in the popular media is when women work in military settings.

As women's roles are seen to be closely related to biological reproduction, so the orientation of **their sexuality is assumed to be heterosexual**. Again feminist research has questioned how far such an orientation is supportive of women's health. The fundamentally unequal nature of relationships between men and women means that heterosexual encounters between them entail continuing negotiations over the risks, costs and consequences of such encounters, including pregnancy and childbirth. Such inequalities also entail the reduced visibility and legitimacy of other sexual orientations. As with other socially problematic categorisations, these have been open to being medicalised. Their reduced visibility and legitimacy have implications for the access to health of non-heterosexual groups.

Surveys of attitudes of nurses and doctors, especially in obstetrics, surgery and family practice, have revealed widespread homophobia. Although relationships with doctors and other health professionals are often seen as being dependent on patients' disclosure of intimate facts, lesbian patients are frequently reluctant to identify themselves as such. This lack of trust and comfort in medical relationships has a range of consequences.

Lesbians are more likely to experience isolation during illness and in their later years. Older lesbians are twice as likely as other women to be living alone. They are also more likely to delay in seeking treatment in mainstream facilities if this means separation from their usual sources of support. The medical advice they receive is less likely to be appropriate as problems in disclosure sets limits on holistic assessment. Stresses which many people experience in dealing with illness are heightened if partners' emotional and practical support is excluded from treatment. Lesbians' access to health resources is, in any case, likely to be more limited by their incomes, which are lower than the population average relative to their level of educational qualification.

Questions which assume the primacy of marriage, rather than more neutral enquiries about whether one lives with a spouse or sexual partner, will not readily encourage confidence in an open attitude to sexual orientation. In any case such assumptions may also be seen as marginalising single or divorced women as well as those in retreat from abusive relationships with male partners.

Many lesbians without children have expressed a wish to conceive. They are much less likely to be assisted through any of the medically regulated technologies. On the other hand, attempts to criminalise the use of artificial insemination by donor (AID) by single and lesbian women has failed because of the difficulty of implementing such a law.

Key questions

What problems would you anticipate affecting any assessment of the health needs of people not living in heterosexual partnerships?

Conclusion: Women acting for health

Gender inequalities in health follow from the basic inequality between men and women in most societies. Women's health is greatly affected by the extent and quality of health services available. Gender inequalities in access to services and in the way in which men and women are treated by the health care system have been identified in modern as well as traditional societies. In developing societies emphasis on women's childbearing roles has resulted in early and excessive childbearing, gender preferences discriminate against female children, while women's work exposes them to health hazards and limits opportunities to take time off for health care.

In all societies balancing parental role commitment with a valued occupational role is harder on women, with correspondingly greater adverse health outcomes. Lone mothers in full-time employment with dependent children have been found to have particularly poor psycho-social health. Women, more than men, are more directly exposed to the economic hardship and child care responsibilities of parenthood, pressures which can significantly increase poor health.

However, strategies to eradicate gender inequalities in health must involve efforts to improve the overall status of women. Women's health organisations have sought to empower themselves through community networking and the use of self-help information. Many women's groups have been outspoken on the dilemmas of reproductive technologies and, as Doyal (1995) emphasises, women should not be seen only as passive victims of an oppressive system but have been active health campaigners world wide.

Women, at least, are increasingly seen as having rights to equal opportunities. Such enhanced life chances are not equally accorded to all social groups. Ethnic minorities have the fundamental problem of being seen as outsiders or 'not belonging' in many societies. The difficulties that ethnic groups face in redressing inequalities and their health consequences are what we consider next.

Further reading

Finch, J. (1989) *Family Obligations and Social Change,* Cambridge: Polity Press.
A thought-provoking study of the moral and practical context of family care work.

Miles, A. (1991) *Women, Health and Medicine,* Milton Keynes: Open University Press.
An accessible introduction to women's health issues.

Roberts, H. (ed.) (1990) *Women's Health Counts,* London: Routledge.
A practical guide to information on women's health.

Wilkinson, S. and Kitzinger, C. (eds) (1994) *Women and Health: Feminist Perspectives,* London: Taylor and Francis.
A collection of feminist studies about women's active contributions to health debates.

Chapter 10 Common and Uncommon Cultures

Most modern societies have to deal with issues arising from the variety among peoples which is a consequence of increasing travel and the growth of communications. The concept of **ethnicity** is a useful way to differentiate between people in terms of their cultural heritage. The right to be counted as a member of a community is based on perceptions of shared cultural heritage. However, ideas that some ethnic groups are 'outsiders' may be used to legitimise decisions to exclude them from full citizenship and also to limit their share in the political, economic and health resources of a society.

Race and discrimination

There is a long-held popular belief that people are biologically different in terms of their **race**, but there is no scientific biological foundation for the existence of racial difference. As we discussed in Chapter 7, race is just another means for differentiating between individuals and placing them in distinct social groups. This differentiation being based on those physical characteristics seen as significant in a particular society (Giddens 1997: 212).

Any group of people with shared physical features and a common cultural heritage which is not seen as part of the majority culture may experience discrimination. The nomadic lifestyle of Gypsies, tinkers and 'New Age' travellers hinders their assimilation into a dominant culture. People of Asian or Afro-Caribbean descent share a common experience of racial discrimination because of the colour of their skin. Other ethnic groups may experience discrimination when linked to a history of the domination of people sharing their cultural traits. Within Britain this has applied to Irish people, whose language was largely suppressed and whose religion was used as the basis of discriminatory practices, the consequences of which can still be seen in the politics of Ireland. It has also applied to the Welsh and Scots, whose languages were previously also suppressed.

When everybody in a given population displays similar dominant cultural characteristics, standardised services are provided, with no need to address inequalities or differences. Local variations may even generate differences in service provision which go unremarked. However, when attention is drawn to differences in moral codes, forms of self-provisioning and alternative religious belief systems, these can be exploited by members of majority groups as a reason to censure ethnic minorities. The experience of Jewish people for much of European history offers evidence of this.

Given the political and economic influences which stimulated travel, cultural differences are often characterised by relationships of domination between peoples, communities and societies. Anthony Smith (1986, 1991) has pointed to the importance of ethnicity in the establishment of national identity, so a divisive or non-inclusive history may play a central part in people's cultural heritage. It may provide the basis for a complex of moral, economic and legislative structures which assign or deny rights of access to respect, to residence and to scarce economic and political resources. Activities of inclusion and exclusion may be justified with references to visible cultural markers such as appearance, skin colour or dress, religious beliefs and practices, and language. Discrimination can be as mundane as the pink-skin colour of sticking plasters.

Mass immigration has been actively encouraged from other societies at times when developing economies have required labour. Groups who have been targeted have often been those with less organised protection of their pay and working conditions. Invited immigration only takes place when newcomers are not seen as a serious political threat by majority groups. In the long term all marginalised groups will experience persistently higher rates of unemployment and other material and health disadvantages.

Expressing cultural preferences in aspects of everyday living, including health care, is therefore neither trivial nor easy. More powerful groupings of the dominant culture can enforce their own preferences. It may be possible for them to resist or suppress the cultural preferences of individuals who are not members of the dominant groups. **Patterns of social activity which base exclusion on ethnic difference constitute the core of racism.**

Race and ethnicity cannot be treated simply as forms of difference. Their consistent links with claims to dominance require us to see them as further bases for socially structured inequality. Controversies about immigration often raise fears about how far new ethnic groups can be assimilated. Such questions are often posed by groups who perceive their local or international dominance as under threat. Discussions of ethnic differences and rights have therefore often been linked to views that the ethnically differentiated 'belong' somewhere else. As the groups continue to engage in their normal cultural practices they can be conveniently stereotyped as being unwilling to 'fit in', holding political allegiances outside the locality or country, taking local economic resources elsewhere or fragmenting local cultures and communities.

Exercise

Find a recent newspaper article discussing an issue focused on an individual or group identified as ethnically distinct.

Would you characterise this individual or group as belonging to 'the majority ethnic group' or 'a minority'?

In what ways does the tone of the article suggest that traits associated with the ethnic identity of the individual or group are desirable or undesirable, healthy or unhealthy?

Does the newspaper's discussion of this individual or group offer comment on their rights to resources or residence within this society?

Networks and ghettos

In the USA, where there have been many waves of immigration, predictions were made earlier in the twentieth century that society would prove to be a 'melting pot' for multicultural assimilation. These predictions were based on the assumption that the children of migrant parents would or should adopt the language and customs of the host communities, eventually blending indistinguishably with them. However, ethnically distinct communities persisted. These were often seen as ghetto communities, taking the image of the earlier enclaves of Jewish communities in Europe, which remained culturally and geographically distinct and which frequently experienced social and political disadvantages.

Initial investigations from an interactionist theoretical perspective explained such persistence through the determination of community members to preserve their ethnicity. Their continuing community membership was important for gaining trade and economic partnerships, marriage partners and family support. However, the right to such ethnic community-based resources may require individuals to provide proof of their continuing community loyalty in their use of language, religious activities and public social relationships. These are sometimes called **'pull' explanations**, that is, ethnic ties of identity which pull communities together.

'Push' explanations have also been advanced. These point to ways in which structural features of the wider society, or the resistance of dominant groups, can generate barriers to the attempts of ethnic minorities to gain equal resources or acceptance. In this way external social processes can underline ethnic difference by devaluing or attempting to suppress cultural differences which minorities find impossible to abandon. They may then establish and sustain alternative networks to provide access to resources such as jobs, housing or financial credit (Suttles 1972).

Another external influence is the market downgrading of some occupations. Jobs which do not offer pay or conditions acceptable to members of dominant ethnic groups may be sought by other ethnic groupings. There are usually higher rates of ethnic minority employment in domestic and public cleaning, and transport jobs. Other ethnic **niche occupations** include taxi work, the clothing industry, building work, specialist grocery shops and catering. Such work may originate in community self-provisioning for specific items of cultural consumption and may characteristically draw on family and other informal contacts to obtain and maintain work.

Marginalisation

Higher levels of socio-economic disadvantages are especially encountered by black ethnic groups. Racism fosters beliefs which perpetuate patterns of disadvantage. Racial prejudice involves the exploitation of those groups who are the subject of racism and operates at both individual and structural levels of society. Visibly different ethnic behaviour threatens majority groups, who feel unable to employ traditional informal mechanisms of control which rely on general social agreements about 'usual behaviour'. We discussed this in Chapter 3 when looking at roles, relationships and social expectations. When conditions of scarcity exist in a society, groups under pressure seek to link their problems to outsiders.

Possible social sanctions include stereotyping marginalised groups to stigmatise them as bringers of trouble. Stereotypes of ethnic minority groups may even link specific disease epidemics to immigration, further justifying their isolation. There is no evidence to support such a view. In poorer occupational classes in the UK British-born men have higher mortality rates than men born in India, Pakistan or the West Indies. Most immigrant groups have lower mortality rates than those in their countries of birth, but this may be because healthier than average individuals have selected themselves for immigration.

The epidemiological picture is more complicated than it appears. In the UK all immigrant groups have been found to have a higher than average mortality from tuberculosis and accidents, but a lower than average one from diseases such as bronchitis (Benzeval *et al.* 1995). Immigrants from the Indian subcontinent have low mortality from several cancers which are common in Britain. However, they suffer higher rates of mortality from liver cancer, strokes, heart disease and diabetes. Some ethnic groups may be subject to specific congenital diseases, such as thalassaemia or sickle cell anaemia.

This still does not fit simple stereotypes about black immigrants bringing diseases with them. They may well be at risk, however, from the social and economic conditions they encounter within the host society and which are heightened within racist settings. The social consequences of racial inequality could be much more powerful determinants of the health status of ethnic minority groups than are genetic or culturally endowed traits.

The concept of **social networks** is helpful for understanding how social groups organise their responses to structural pressures. A social network is the system of ongoing relationships in which individuals are involved, and we discussed their importance in connection with families and households in Chapter 4. The pattern of such relationships may be based on different structures of interaction and communication. Such structures, in turn, influence how an individual connects with other groups and the wider society. Important dimensions of networks include:

- how many people are in direct contact with an individual and how often;
- whether these contacts are based on only one type of social activity (such as employment) or range across several types (including religious activities, family activities and neighbouring);
- levels of everyday local involvement with groups compared with more distant contacts maintained by telephone, mail or long-distance journeys;
- the number of contacts of an individual who are also in contact with each other.

Networks of informal relationships may be crucial to gaining access to material or emotional resources for a socially disadvantaged individual. Morris (1989) has examined how differences in the language and culture of people in North Wales, where a majority of people have Welsh as their birth language, can lead to the development of social support networks very different in size, density and intensity. She found that those individuals who did not build Welsh language and cultural links were more likely to experience social isolation and to feel excluded from a wide range of local community activities.

Wenger (1994) has demonstrated how differences in network types can generate specific patterns of problems presented by older people to helping agencies. Differences between network types are shown to result in different interventions which produce different outcomes. Some interventions will not work with some types of network. Sensitivity to differences in support networks will help in understanding what an individual's network is likely to provide, what help it is likely to need and the most efficient types of intervention.

> **Exercise**
>
> Make a list of cultural activities which you have personally experienced and through which you think social networks may be sustained – things like a sports or social club, or a cafe or bar you go to regularly. How far do these activities call for:
>
> - a particular level of income, skill or language ability;
> - other kinds of cultural knowledge;
> - other 'membership' qualifications?

These other membership qualifications call into question how easily these activities could include an individual with a different skin colour, a different religious background or a different language from yourself – or even one who wears distinctively different clothes, jewellery or facial adornment.

Approaches to illness and life events

In any society birth and death are special social events because social groupings and networks have to be adjusted to take account of the resulting changes. At birth new members are being added, with all the implications this has for how people are related and what is owed to and expected of new members of the group. At a death many relationships and groupings may be transformed or even broken. You only have to think of the consequences for families of the death of a member who has always made traditional family gatherings, such as Christmas, 'special' in order to bring the family together as a group. Specific social roles may need to be taken up or reallocated. All these readjustments in relationships have to be made in terms of the kinds of expectation the groups involved already have of each other. These combine moral beliefs and expectations about what ought to happen within relationships, based on individual and community life histories. This clarifies why people do not necessarily act or react in the same way, especially at the time of birth and death.

Within some communities there are strongly held moral expectations of how members should behave. We may have convictions about 'what should be done' or 'what is right' at a time when people from other ethnic backgrounds might respond equally strongly but with different ways of ordering their experiences. This can lead to unfortunate misunderstandings and failures on the part of health professionals to appreciate which kinds of support may be most appropriate in which context. It may even lead to people from backgrounds different from those of the health professional being stigmatised or sanctioned for behaving 'unnaturally'. This could be as direct as what counts as an appropriate display of emotion – of fear or of grief.

Differences in moral beliefs are bound up with practical religious differences. Religious organisations are providers of support and networking which are unavailable from the wider society. Catholic churches are important for Irish and some East European groups, mosques for Asian and African ethnic communities and synagogues for Jewish people. They may be vital providers of educational and welfare services, health guidance and employment contacts.

Religious buildings and festivals provide important gathering points for a wide range of communal activities, and religious leaders often act as community spokespeople. Fundamentalist revivals in both Christian and Islamic religious activities have especially emphasised the renewal of community and family support. Noting the diversity of such religious systems is a useful reminder that ethnic minorities cannot be treated as constituting a homogeneous group. Even within communities labelled as Asian or Afro-Caribbean there are wide differences in beliefs, traditions, language and resources. Religious and moral value systems operate as 'pull' factors in creating ethnic communities. However, in the face of a hostile majority, religious and cultural value systems may be used by ethnic minority groups to help confirm the legitimacy of alternative communities.

Times of illness, important life events and issues of fertility may be dealt with through customary or ritual activities, or through religious mediators who help to restore a sense of order over such events. This may mean that community members expect to refer to a range of people whose authority may also be seen as important in managing such events, so that, although health care professionals may be important at such times, the primacy of their authority cannot be taken for granted. Concepts other than medical ones should be considered in addressing socially important issues such as celebrations of birth or bereavement ceremonies. Collective preparations may be made; particular foods may be especially valued or avoided. The avoidance of various forms of 'pollution' from specific foods, materials, events or people could be important in cultural terms (Williams and Collins 1995).

Exercise

Think of any recent traditional festival or celebration you have attended: a wedding, christening, birthday or anniversary.

Did it have any religious connotation? If so, how did this affect the place in which it was held and which people took part?

Were any special foods expected?

Who prepared or supplied these?

What role were particular families or family members expected to play?

Many varieties of cultural practices are found in how festivals are conducted. Even within the dominant culture there are subcultural variations – not everyone celebrates a birthday in the same way. Ethnic minority groups may adhere more rigorously to traditional practices as a way of reasserting their special identity. Compare your experiences with those of colleagues and friends. Look closely at such details as social roles, language used and clothes worn.

Multiculturalism and 'moral decline'

Fears of moral decline or uncertainty in multicultural, pluralist societies are often associated with a perceived loss of ethnic supremacy. This may be symbolically expressed using **disease imagery** or **notions of moral pollution**. It could be argued that a society apparently secure in its moral values may also be one in which dominant groups are also secure. The challenges offered by ethnic diversity can generate moral outrage on the part of such groups.

Alternative family structures amplify the nature of the perceived threat. Ethnic variations in family structure offer a challenge to the dominant conventions of kinship connections, inheritance and distributions of power in households. The variety of family and household types may include polygamy, cousin marriage, matriarchal households, authority of uncles rather than fathers, arranged marriages and divorce by public statement rather than in secular courts.

It can be argued that multiculturalism does not so much mean that moralities are being diluted but that the complexity of moral codes must be recognised. Such an approach would acknowledge the existence of multiple belief systems and question the dominance of any single social group. Less moral certainty could be beneficial for opposing bigotry and prejudice. This would fit with postmodernist debates about social differences and power. Moral and cultural relativism does not necessarily produce a moral vacuum.

Community self-care

Shared activities within households, providing informal support for care, constitute the networks which form the basis of community self-care. Within many Western industrial societies there are widespread assumptions that such responsibilities fall on the nuclear family, with varying degrees of state support. Other societies highlight the greater responsibilities taken by extended family networks. In the context of Western societies it is often assumed that ethnic minority group members are both unwilling to seek public service support, and self-sufficient in terms of resources in their family and community-based networks. This ignores ways in which ethnic minority groups are often additionally disadvantaged in terms of access to care support and medical treatment.

Rather than ethnic minority groups being self-sufficient, it is more likely that social isolation and economic disadvantage make self-care and family care difficult for such groups. Whatever their cultural preferences, ethnic groups are unlikely to be able to sustain long-term health care in a context of socio-economic pressure. Language and cultural differences or racial discrimination can obstruct access to health care resources.

Where ethnic groups use a non-majority language and where social organisation focuses women's activities in the home, women are less likely to speak the majority language. This may make it more difficult to obtain treatment or health advice. Within Britain there is little systematic provision of translation or interpreting services except where legislation has been passed to support minority languages. As language issues are not seen as strictly medical priorities, health services language initiatives are sporadic.

Cultural barriers are especially problematic since addressing them calls for care workers and managers from majority ethnic groups to recognise that other cultural practices should be acknowledged. These include expectations within some communities that individuals should receive personal care and medical consultations from people of the same sex. Expectations of what constitutes a 'proper' meal are integral to culture. Advice on fertility treatment, family planning and the prevention of sexually transmitted diseases may need to take account of very specific community expectations of how such topics may be discussed. The implications of such expectations are clear when we think about how care services may need to be planned for older people, whether in their own homes or in residential home care.

Exercise

Think about any long-stay residential care home of which you have had experience.

What evidence do you have that it caters for differences in:

● language?

● cultural background (choice of food, communal events)?

● religion?

Can you think of any local ethnic minority group which does not have older members in this home?

What issues do you think might arise for such an individual who came to live in this home?

Racial discrimination may affect health chances through the effects of structural socio-economic inequalities experienced by ethnic groups. However, discriminatory effects may also be seen in stereotyping. This may, in turn, be used to justify services omitting any specific assessments of their needs or to tailor community provision. Individual assessment would allow needs to be identified where resources are not available in practice to individual members of specific ethnic groups. These may be compounded by failures to facilitate accurate interpretation of language or interaction. Health services respond very unsystematically to such needs. In order to guarantee equal access to all groups, care agencies need to improve their awareness of where routes to care may need to be structured differently to take account of the different support networks in ethnic communities. A collective assessment process would recognise the role of majority group practices or dynamics in the wider society in creating patterns of health problems linked to ethnic minority group membership.

Informal networks are important in providing advice on health, in giving health care and in supporting individuals in decisions about when to consult official health services. However, ethnic minority groups are much less likely to find health advisors from similar cultural and class backgrounds, except through lay or traditional networks.

To improve awareness we must look beyond simplistic notions of one community sharing ethnic and socio-economic characteristics. Ethnic and class groupings may as easily cut across as reinforce communities. This is seen in multiracial tensions between many urban communities, often expressed in conflict over the allocation of welfare, housing and health provision. Divisive community dynamics in these situations can lead to persistent and violent racial harassment. In some cases local pressures bring about local alliances of diverse groups co-operating across ethnic divides. They have taken action over drugs, traffic problems, housing or environmental issues (Braithwaite and Lythcott 1989).

In addition to expressing different needs, the existence of multi-ethnic groups adds to a society's awareness of the variety of forms in which care can be provided. This has had an impact in the proliferation of complementary and alternative forms of medicine such as acupuncture, homeopathy, herbalism and reflexology. Such health care practices are gradually being incorporated into mainstream areas of medical care. One example is massage, which is an integral part of baby care in many parts of India and is increasingly used in palliative care to relieve stress and pain.

Medical traditions

A combination of issues of access and of community values and customs shapes the treatment options available to different ethnic groups. Many ethnic groups have long standing traditions of medicine. In India, for example, there are alternative systems of medicine which run in parallel. Ayurvedic medicine is the most commonly used, but alongside allopathic medicine. In Western societies such systems are likely to be seen as complementary medicines at best or possibly not given any medical status.

The degree to which ethnic group members use mainstream Western medicine could be seen as an index not only of their communities' assimilation, but also of their social class status. Poorer sections of Asian communities often use herbal remedies. Middle-class sections of the same communities are almost wholly reliant on Western forms of medicine. Afro-Caribbean people are more likely to use herbal remedies. Women in both communities are more likely to use herbal remedies. Such remedies provide additional resources in conditions of scarcity. However, they are also likely to be associated with a continuation of traditional belief systems and networks.

These factors shape the responses of different ethnic group members to medical interventions. In some contexts Western medicine may be distrusted if it contradicts important aspects of cultural identity and may be seen as the 'alternative' to traditional remedies. In such cases medical interventions will not be viewed by members as long-term treatment options. If treatments are seen as interfering with normal lifestyles, patients may be reluctant to maintain them. For example, a drugs regime to counteract hypertension may be seen as too debilitating. Responses like this can contradict doctors' expectations of compliance and may run counter to their ideas about how 'good patients' should behave (Culley 1996).

High rates of serious mental illness are recorded among all black minority groups. The reasons for this have been the subject of controversy, over whether such rates reflect biological differences, the outcome of social pressures or simply cultural biases in the diagnostic methods used by psychiatrists. Given the links between belief and value systems and the interpretation of behaviour already discussed, it is difficult to be confident that diagnostic categories in mental health are comparable across cultures. The more holistic approach of Littlewood and Lipsedge

(1989) explains individuals' experiences of contrasting cultures. Mental illness becomes a way of symbolically representing power inequality, misfortune and an attempt to adjust to contradictory value systems.

Within the wider population there are links between mental ill health and problems with employment and housing. Where ethnic disadvantages in these areas are encountered, such stresses will be more likely. Within Afro-Caribbean communities behavioural problems and mental illness are often more visible and more likely to be regulated through police action. Young people from these communities are more likely to be excluded from conventional education, to be sent to special schools and to be charged with delinquency.

Within the mental health system there is evidence of discrimination. Black patients diagnosed as suffering from psychoses are twice as likely as white patients – including white immigrants – to be detained involuntarily. They are more likely to receive prescriptions of electroconvulsive therapy and psychotropic drugs rather than the gentler forms of care such as 'talking therapies'. Many individual and group therapies are based on the exercise of particular communicative skills as well as middle-class cultural practices which encourage the discussion of feelings. The kinds of ethnic difference we have discussed make it less likely that members of ethnic minority groups will be seen as meeting the criteria for such therapies.

For both physical and mental illnesses there is evidence that structural factors, rather than lifestyle or genetics, determine racial disadvantages, including health and health care problems. As with gender, medicalisation of some of the socio-economic problems of ethnic groups may be one response by the wider society. That is to say, such problems may be defined as having medical causes and solutions. If their causes lie beyond the medical, and if medical interventions are to be used effectively, it may be necessary to define them more flexibly and in combination with other kinds of activity.

Yet health professionals, in common with any majority group behaviour, may still be prone to blame the 'different'. Patients may be seen as 'time wasting' if their complaints are viewed as being outside the competence of health professionals. Particular treatments may be seen by patients from some ethnic groups as depriving them of traditions without offering much in return (Morgan 1996).

Ethnic minority communities sometimes counteract failures to recognise their needs by identifying their own needs and by lobbying, or refuse co-operation if appropriate services are not developed. Ethnic minority groups are more likely to be employed in less well paid jobs in health care, reducing the chances that their needs and values will be reflected in health services decision-making structures. Where health service managers are insulated from user pressure, ethnic minority groups will need to gain knowledge of decision-making structures in order to provoke more response.

Exercise

What kinds of communication activity are called for in gaining treatment for:

● a stomach upset;

● persistent headaches;

● arthritis;

● panic attacks;

● fertility problems?

In what ways do you think success in obtaining satisfactory treatment may be affected:

● if your family does not share the majority ethnic background;

● if your first language is not the majority language?

Think beyond the immediate communication channels of language and roles. Remember how important your other senses, such as smell, touch and vision, are. How are such senses differently employed within and between different cultures?

Conclusion

There is debate about whether racial disadvantages exist that are independent of class disadvantages. The material problems of ethnic difference are closely linked to the location of individuals within the occupational structure. It is argued that, as some ethnic minority groups appear to be better placed within the class structure than most of the majority population, this disproves the notion of a separate racial disadvantage. However, as with arguments about gender or age, we must not assume that ethnic differences are homogeneous. A diversity of ethnic experience should be recognised, which is sometimes cut across by local and class factors.

One approach is to see ethnic groups as trapped in a **race-based underclass**, but the complexity of such a concept can be seen in the advocacy for it from both conservative and liberal political traditions (Murray 1984, Field 1989) and the total opposition toward the idea from others (Mann 1992). However, the weight of historical, political and economic evidence suggests that discrimination based on race genuinely contributes to multiple disadvantages. A clear awareness of these ethnic dimensions is required for effective health support.

In these last three chapters we have discussed how class, gender and ethnic differences directly affect people's beliefs and behaviour with regard to health and caring, but beliefs and behaviour are also influenced by many other factors. In Chapter 11 we will consider some other sources of influence on health-related practices.

Further reading

Ahmad, W.I.U. (ed.) (1993) *Race and Health in Contemporary Britain*, Buckingham: Open University Press.
A collection of articles offering a summary of key issues.

Gilroy, P. (1987) *There Ain't no Black in the Union Jack*, London: Hutchinson.
A lively discussion of how black people have been marginalised in the UK.

Norman, A. (1985) *Triple Jeopardy: Growing Old in a Second Homeland*, London: Centre for Policy on Ageing.
A study of how problems of ageing are compounded by racism.

Sheldon, T.S. and Parker, H. (1992) 'Race and ethnicity in health research', *Journal of Public Medicine*, **14**: 104–10.
A useful review of research on race and health.

Chapter 11 Beliefs, Moralities and Ideologies of Care

People hold a range of everyday ideas about why we stay healthy and what makes us ill. These are known as 'lay' concepts or models of health and illness. Professionals also possess more detailed 'expert' models and concepts. There is inevitably a mix of lay and expert models in both perspectives. Professionals are, after all, also people with particular cultural background influences and experiences, and non-professionals are not ignorant of complex reasons for illness and health.

We trust that professionals' knowledge is based more on **systematically researched evidence** (science) and upon their collective experience of favourable treatment procedures. There is, however, little doubt that lay social and cultural concepts do play a part in the professionals' views of illness and treatment. In previous chapters we have encouraged professional health carers to address their own prejudices, stereotypes and ideologies about the causes of health and illness.

Accounting for health and illness

We gain access to people's beliefs and conceptual models through **discourse**, the reasons for health and illness that they put forward in conversation. Rarely are such accounts comprehensive: they permit only a partial glimpse of the broader ideology upon which any particular account is based. Accounts vary according to the situation in which they are offered. They are used to manipulate and manage situations, to reveal or to conceal those beliefs which individuals think relevant. Health and illness accounts are based on views about the human body in general, an individual's own body and ideas about natural and normal phenomena.

On the whole we see illness as a 'bad thing' which we wish to eradicate, and health as a 'good thing' which we wish to establish and maintain. There are times, however, when illness can be evaluated positively and health negatively. Thus illness may sometimes be seen as a way to force someone to take much needed rest, while an excessive concern with healthy eating may be seen as obsessive or neurotic.

Exercise

Write down the word for an aspect of your own behaviour which you consider to be 'healthy'.

Write down why you think it healthy and why you continue to engage in that behaviour.

Also write down any behaviour you engage in which you think is healthy but which others have told you is unhealthy, and why they say it is unhealthy.

Your own and others' discourse contains many hidden assumptions about the causes of ill health. Return to your answers to these questions as you read through this chapter and consider the lay models being adopted.

As we explained in Chapter 3 social order depends upon people fulfilling routine expectations. Health is treated as a normal state of physical and mental well-being. Departures from health become a focus for concern if they interfere with normal social interaction. In recent years health has become less taken for granted and regarded as something to be accomplished with some thought and effort. Questioning the causes of health is usually provoked when we lose it.

Lay models of illness vary widely between and within cultures, but Chrisman (1977) has grouped them into four basic types of cause:

- **invasion from outside** – a germ, cancer, something eaten, an intruding object or evil spirits;
- **degeneration within** – the body becoming run down, toxic or wearing out;
- **mechanical defects** – a blockage or internal organ malfunction;
- **balance problems** – flaws in the diet or nutrition, taking inadequate sleep or rest, missing harmony in life and human relations.

Stainton Rogers (1991) has identified common features of acceptable explanations for illness. Similarly, Radley (1994) has outlined patterns in the experience of illness which help us to make sense of it. Both lay and professional models of illness must address each of the following components:

1. **identification** – awareness of and labelling of the illness;
2. **symptomatology** – recognition of symptoms and the mode of onset;
3. **aetiology** – postulated causes of the condition;
4. **pathophysiology** – long- and short-term consequences, the abnormal nature of the condition and its likely outcomes;
5. **course of sickness** – the experience of the illness, the 'time line', duration, severity, periodicity (acute, cyclic or chronic) and sick role behaviour;
6. **treatment/therapy** – the nature and experience of treatment.

Both professionals and clients use these criteria to interpret symptoms, to make choices between available therapies and therapists, and to give meaning to the experience of sickness and treatment. Lay constructs and expert medical models share many features in relation to appropriate categories into which causes and consequences must fit. Some interaction between popular understanding and authoritative scientific explanations is bound to take place as health research findings are disseminated via the popular media.

> **Exercise**
>
> Think of a range of recent examples of illness which you have witnessed or experienced.
>
> How did your accounts, or the accounts of others, relate to these models of illness?
>
> What sorts of explanation were put forward by others?
>
> What sorts of explanation did you find acceptable?
>
> In what circumstances were explanations not sought?

Levels of explanation

Rarely do we take accounts at face value. People offer accounts according to particular circumstances. Medical professionals believe that some explanations are more valid than others. Lay accounts are at the bottom of their hierarchy, and scientifically validated explanations are at the top. It need not matter in practice if a common-sense explanation is unscientific so long as it improves health. Some pregnant women give up smoking because they believe that it pollutes the soul rather than because they believe the scientific evidence that it pollutes their own body and that of their fetus (Adler *et al.* 1992). As Douglas (1992) points out it is for this sort of reason that magic survives in traditional societies. It appears to work for those who believe it and practise it. This kind of observation justifies professionals offering patients only partial explanations of their illness and treatment. It may seem patronising and as further subordinating the patient, but is excused on the grounds that excess detail may be confusing or induce anxiety.

Everyday and scientific explanations

Scientific explanations lead to objective generalisations called **laws**. A law offers a means of systematically and consistently predicting patterns of precisely defined and measurable events. The status of scientific explanations depends upon meeting the requirements of logic and **formal standards of adequacy** for an explanation. Everyday explanations have ordinary social standards of acceptability. However, even science can be seen as merely another means of constructing socially agreed terms and frameworks. What are seen as 'facts', 'events', 'truth' and 'logic' are all negotiated between scientists in particular kinds of social interaction.

Anthropologists in the early twentieth century typically distinguished between **primitive** and **civilised medical systems**. Primitive concepts have been seen as irrational when based on religious superstitions. Modern medicine, in contrast, is assumed to be based on rational science and the logical exploration of observable evidence. However, **clinical effectiveness** initiatives and pleas for the growth of **evidence-based health care** in recent years have demonstrated just how little medical practice has been based on rigorous scientific research. Estimates suggest that less than 20 per cent of medical practice has been validated in systematic inquiry: much clinical practice went on without the rigorous proof assumed to be vital for adequate scientific explanation. Clinical work was seen as effective and so was used because it appeared to be successful. The same criterion is adopted to assess the success of magic.

More recently, writers such as Payer (1990) have argued that all societies' systems of medicine and medical explanation must be set in a broader cultural and ecological context. Some social scientists have actually used concepts applied to the study of very different societies to ask how far we can take for granted the forms of explanation accepted in our own. For example, Douglas (1973) uses ideas about ritual, taboo and pollution to make us think differently about our notions of dirt, infection and disease. The difference between everyday and scientific explanation may be more a matter of degree than of kind. Scientists are more systematic and more selective in accounting for their explanations, but this is not to say that their reasoning methods are very different from those of everyday life.

Scientific status does more than enhance the adequacy of an explanation; it gives authority to the users of such explanations. Medical practitioners are seen as having the expertise to offer effective treatment and are therefore accorded the social status and resources which give them more credibility. To be effective their explanatory accounts must be seen as in some way superior to everyday explanations.

This should not mean that medical judgements and actions cannot be questioned. Gabe *et al.* (1994) add to a lengthy tradition which questions whether the assumed superiority of medical accounts has been taken too far. The power accruing to medical practitioners as a particular social grouping is seen in the ways our lives have been increasingly **medicalised**:

- in the details of our private lives – diet, exercise, sex and even emotion and expression;
- in public life – for example, constraining the advertising of drugs and alcohol;
- in extending technical control – over who can prescribe drugs and medical procedures such as kidney transplants, IVF or genetic engineering;
- in gaining dominance of taboo areas – such as alcohol use and child abuse.

The accounts and understandings of lower-status groups become generally discounted not only by medical specialists, but also by those groups themselves. Lay people may find it difficult to take their own understandings of the world seriously.

We need to examine more closely how we derive our ideas about health from our ideas of what is seen as normal in everyday life. Normal people are healthy, and healthy people are normal; there is a great deal of moral pressure not to be seen as odd, unnatural or abnormal. This provides strong incentives to develop socially acceptable explanations about how and why we become ill.

Other explanations for abnormalities which were once acceptable, such as witchcraft or sin, are now less valid. When our normal life experiences are biologically disturbed, illness is now the main explanation for behaving in unusual ways. As we discussed in Chapter 3 we do expect people who are ill to remove themselves from public life. Thus illness behaviour is not entirely immune from guilt, blame and shame (Finerman and Bennett 1995).

Permanent illness and disability may be highly stigmatising. Where life-threatening illnesses such as AIDS cannot be socially ignored, they may be seen as morally threatening plagues associated with subgroups in society. The moral panic which surrounds attitudes to some illnesses and the explanations of their causes reveals the connection between illness accounts and a wider moral order. We pursue this in more detail in Chapter 12.

> **Exercise**
>
> Study one illness in detail:
>
> Why might rheumatoid arthritis patients try to 'cover up and keep up'?
>
> How easy is this, given the nature of rheumatoid symptoms?
>
> How likely are medical staff to find out about such patients' problems in coping?
>
> What might this mean for official records about the condition?

The symptoms of pain, immobility and fatigue associated with rheumatoid arthritis vary daily. Sufferers find it difficult to predict how they will carry out tasks which sustain their independence and self-esteem. This makes it important to cover up symptoms and keep up appearances of normality. The effort of sustaining this produces further fatigue. It also makes it more difficult for them to discuss their coping strategies with medical staff who they feel do not fully understand or accept their accounts of what is important about their illness.

Attitudes to the body

The effectiveness of treatment and scientific enquiry about the causes of illness have depended upon common-sense under-standings of the nature of the human body. The early problems faced by anatomists over the dissection of corpses offer a graphic example of religious beliefs obstructing progress. The body is now commonly seen as a combination of biological, anatomical, physiological and spiritual entities and processes which interact within a social and physical environment.

The most common assumption about bodies and minds is that some are 'able' and others are not. The able/disabled distinction is one that needs to be added to the list of sources of structured inequality which we have already discussed. Healthy individuals are assumed to have no bodily or mental disadvantages and constitute the norm. The **'dis-abled' body and mind is effectively excluded from normal social intercourse**. Instead of providing for degrees of blindness, deafness, learning deficiency and physical incapacity, our society should assume that there are widely varying degrees of visual acuity, hearing, learning ability and physical capability among the population. It is only relatively recently that urban spaces have been designed to take account of the 'abilities' of the full range of potential users of that space.

Exercise

Write about your views of your own body.

What are your special physical attributes?

Is there anything about your body you are unhappy with? Why?

What pleases or displeases you about other people's bodies and what they do with them? Why?

Why do we distinguish between public and private parts of the body?

Attitudes toward our own bodies and prejudices about other people's bodies reveal a great deal about assumptions of the ideal, of normality and of what it means to be able-bodied.

Blame and responsibility: attributing motives and causes

The need to explain health and illness more rigorously confronts us all when we are ill or when someone dear to us is ill or even dying. It is hard to be dispassionate under such conditions, and many of our hidden assumptions about health and illness are revealed when we seek to apportion blame. Blaming takes place when we believe illness to be caused by a person or people rather than being a random natural occurrence. Blame is a probable element in the illness accounts of both experts and the lay public.

Health professionals evidently make attributions of control and blame for illness which vary according to their attitudes towards patients and their knowledge of the disorder or complaint. As Sharu (1996) argues this may have consequences for the quality of care and the degree of empathy and sympathy which carers give to their client.

People sometimes see themselves as responsible for their own illness on the grounds of some divine retribution for a sinful action committed earlier in life. More often than not people can see themselves as responsible for the onset of illness and lack of health as a result of action they took or neglected to take. Forms of self-abuse could include smoking, eating and drinking to excess or promiscuity, while self-neglect might occur with a poorly chosen diet or with deferring medical treatment. As Weiner (1993) suggests a distinction between sin and sickness is vital to the attribution of personal responsibility and blame.

Family members can be blamed for illness as a consequence of conscious abuse or neglect. More frequently, families have to bear responsibility for hereditary factors or a lack of knowledge about healthy living. Blame is often placed on a range of generalised others such as 'the system', the health services and the medical profession, or charges of specific abuse or neglect may be made against named practitioners.

If no humans or forms of human organisation can be blamed, a search for physiological causes is deemed appropriate (Peterson 1995). Such causes are viewed as the outcome of chance or nature. Illness is part of the natural order, humans cannot avoid it and, if they are unlucky, they become ill.

More challenging issues about allocating responsibility come when accounting for death. Coroners point out how a description by a medical practitioner of why someone died must include a full 'natural history' for the death. If a medical practitioner cannot decide and offer an acceptable cause of death, then, by law, it becomes a coroner's case. Thus old age is not an officially acceptable cause of death in the UK. Practitioners are discouraged from putting 'old age' as the sole cause of death on a death certificate. It is seen as slightly more acceptable if the dead person is aged seventy or over.

It has often been pointed out how the medicalisation of certain conditions and the attributions associated with them reveals an underlying acceptance of social order, norms and values. To take one example, infertility is commonly referred to as a 'fault' in one or both partners. This implies blame for the inability to conceive. Yet the couple have only 'failed' to meet cultural expectations for the raising of a family. Becker and Nachtigall (1992) discuss how medicalising infertility stigmatises women who may be seen as defective due to their childlessness. However, this amounts to a reassertion of dominant gender role expectations. Both patient and health care practitioner are colluding in the implication that the inability biologically to reproduce is abnormal and that an illness must therefore exist. There is then pressure on the 'barren' woman to exhaust all possible treatments to ensure reproduction. Yet treatment does not diminish feelings of abnormality: it exacerbates them by the intensity of the pursuit. The practitioner thereby participates in the maintenance of negative cultural attitudes about childlessness.

Blame cannot be easily attributed to innocent victims. The death, illness or handicap of a young child seems unfair to most people. It is assumed that, given their short life and innocence, there can be nothing the child itself could have done wrong. If there is to be any blaming, only adults must bear it. For blame to be attributed to a victim their innocence must become compromised in some way. Variations in illness attribution might thus occur systematically according to modifications of the patient's innocence by association with other acts attached to the patient's nature or character. One can anticipate variations in attribution according to age, gender, being 'too fat' or 'too thin', ethnic cultural practices, risky lifestyles and so on – many of the characteristics on which inequality is based, as already discussed.

The debate over euthanasia illustrates the moral complexities entailed in assigning blame. The key issue here is whether there is a distinction between allowing someone to die and actively assisting their death. Reasons given for the assistance are assessed according to how morally acceptable we hold particular intentions to be.

There are limiting factors in the search for causes of illness. With some issues fear of litigation inhibits the concern to locate causes, even though the identification of non-human causes or the reallocating of blame might alleviate the suffering of relatives or even health care professionals who suspect their own complicity in unfavourable treatment outcomes. Equally, the search for cause might be limited by time and place or by the idea that it took place too long ago to be of concern.

Exercise

Think of an illness or accidental injury that you recently experienced. Conduct a blame analysis by answering these questions:

cont'd

For the accident: 'Who did what to whom, why, when, where and how?'

For an illness: 'What happened, to whom, why, when, where and how?'

Ask other people to give their account of the same illness or accident. Note in which respects the accounts differ, especially with regard to 'cause' and 'blame'. Did the seeking of treatment alone absolve people of any guilt for illness or accident and outcomes? To what extent did the burden of responsibility for favourable outcomes fall on the health care professional?

Taking chances

The contemporary interest in health risks has been an inevitable consequence of concern with blame and responsibility. Fears of adverse reactions to childhood immunisation and the growth of genetic testing and counselling have increased the public awareness of **risk**. Consideration is now being given to the labelling of therapeutic drugs with known 'risk ratings'.

The concept of risk underpins our views on health. How real is our understanding of the chances we are taking with our health when we smoke, drink alcohol to excess, eat too much and so on? Knowing something is good for us, but not attempting to improve our intake or uptake of it is the fundamental problem confronting health education and promotion. Apportioning blame in this case depends on the effective public availability of health knowledge (Gabe 1995).

We do appear to persist with things which are good for us if we believe we can continue to control them without interference from outside. If seeking health lowers the quality of life, people might not think it is worth the effort. We conduct personal cost–benefit analyses of dietary or exercise-related health activities.

Genetic blueprinting suggests an element of fatalism in modern lay conceptions of health and illness: the cards have already been dealt for you and your chances of survival determined. We may feel that there is little we can do about the biological characteristics with which we have been endowed, and it may appear that we can do little to control our own health.

We do make attempts to avoid any guilt for unhealthy behaviour. We excuse exuberance in the young or occasional overindulgence. The infrequency of a 'non-healthy' activity attenuates the guilt and responsibility associated with it, but responsibility and control are not the same thing. Fatalism and making healthy lifestyle choices are not contradictory. People regard some adverse health outcomes as beyond their control but still try to engage in health-promoting behaviour. Some strategies for changing community health behaviour with disadvantaged populations work by requiring the community to accept responsibility for their problems. At the same time this avoids the debilitating effects of self-blame and makes it possible to take responsibility without taking blame (Neighbors *et al.* 1995).

There are many causes 'beyond one's control' which may give rise to negative outcomes, and outcomes are not always entirely dependent upon intentions. The excessive bearing of blame could become a disincentive to taking responsibility. It is for such reasons that health care professionals have recently been trying to ensure that they do not do everything for their client, and clients have been encouraged to participate in clinical decisions.

Exercise

Write down the word or phrase for an aspect of your own behaviour which you consider to be 'unhealthy'.

Write down why you think it unhealthy.

Write down why you continue to engage in that behaviour.

Consider how much control you have over whether you choose to engage in this behaviour. Who or what else would you see as sharing responsibility for this behaviour?

Conclusion

It is vital to health- and illness-related behaviour to understand how and why attributions change and can be modified. On a clinical level a degree of congruence between patient and practitioner explanatory models might be essential to effective treatment. Incongruence in vital areas affects adherence to treatment, so ways to increase the health professional's awareness of patients' explanatory models need to be studied. The importance of this is evident in how the kinds of explanation that can be given to children affects their willingness to undergo treatment.

Preventing illness and encouraging health depends upon identifying and controlling the causes of ill health. If a physiological cause can be identified, patients will more easily accept a medical intervention. However, it is clear that for some conditions and for some cultures and subcultures, as we discussed in Chapter 10, only certain ways of accounting for illness will be accepted. The health professional's role might then be to offer a rationale for treatment which is acceptable to the patient and which is in the patient's interest, but professionals regularly face the dilemma of acting in the interests of public health or, more narrowly, in their own interests. How much time can be spent explaining things to patients or listening carefully to patients' explanations? Can professionals honestly act in the interests of patients whose behaviour and attitudes are likely to pose a threat to the health and safety of others?

In the last analysis attributions of blame and responsibility will, inevitably, lie with the health care professional. Given the scarcity of health resources, limitations on expertise and the gamut of moral constraints on practice, health professionals routinely take treatment decisions which reassert the broader structural inequalities of the society in which they are operating. Resources are limited, yet they still need to be allocated. How can they ever be fairly distributed among those seeking care and support?

Exercise

As a final exercise in this chapter:

What were/are your motives for becoming a health professional?

cont'd

> What do you believe to be your primary function/major role as a
> health care practitioner?

Issues of blame, moral responsibility, power and control come
together in the answer to such questions. For example, does your
professional 'calling' result in allegiances owed to colleagues or
clients or the health of the nation or public order? How far can
these potentially contradictory obligations be balanced? After
answering this question, look back and compare how you
answered a similar question in the Preface at the start of the book.

Beliefs about what constitutes bad health have strong moral
connotations. The pressure to medicalise some aspects of human
behaviour is related to the need to control behaviour or attitudes
considered deviant or unhealthy. In Chapter 12 we consider
why and how society attempts to control some illnesses and
treat some socially deviant behaviour as if it were an illness-
related 'condition'.

Further reading

Backett, K. (1992) 'Taboos and excesses: lay health moralities in middle
class families', *Sociology of Health and Illness*, **14**: 255–74.
Blaxter, M. (1983) 'The cause of disease: women talking', *Social Science and
Medicine*, **17**: 59–69.
These articles distinguish between class and gender influences on lay
models of health.

Ewles, L. and Simnett, I. (1992) *Health Promotion – a Practical Guide*,
London: Scutari Press.
The practical angle raises the problem of getting people to accept
rationales for health and illness other than their own.

Radley, A. (ed.) (1993) *Worlds of Illness: Biographical and Cultural Perspectives on Health and Disease*, London: Routledge.
Considers a range of alternative explanations for the experience of
illness.

Thorne, S.E. (1993) *The Social Context of Chronic Illness*, London: Sage.
Attempts to locate illness experiences socially.

Chapter 12   Controlling Conditions

Becoming ill, acquiring a disability or caring for the ill may lead to various **exclusions** and marginalisation from some groups in society and to **inclusion** in others. It is important to understand how the lives and experiences of some people come to be marginalised. The processes by which social deviations are controlled may also provide means of justifying and reinforcing continuing inequalities of opportunity and of power.

Cause and reaction

Sociologists are concerned to understand why things appear to go wrong in society. Why do people commit crimes? What makes people take drugs or deface walls? Why are some people homeless or alcoholic, and why do others commit suicide? Indeed, why are some people sick while others remain healthy? These questions are all about why some people deviate from social standards which are seen as normal.

There is a difference between the causes of problems (**aetiology**) and the influences on our **reactions** to them. Sociology may not have all the aetiological answers since, alongside social causes, there may be biological, psychological, neurophysiological, economic and other reasons why deviant events take place. However, sociologists do try to answer the question: 'What causes people to **see** events as deviant or problematic?'

There is difficulty in keeping questions of cause and reaction separate since it is almost impossible to understand events in isolation from the social and cultural context in which they take place. For example, the act of 'taking one's clothes off' is a fundamentally different event depending on whether it is done in private in one's bedroom, on a beach, in a clinical consulting room, in public at a sports event or in a city centre back street at night. The potential causes of the act of deviance are separate from the various ways in which the **socio-cultural context** of the deviant act influences our perspectives on it. It is for this reason that Howard Becker (1963) pointed out that **no act is inherently deviant**; what makes it deviant is whether society deems it so.

Social perspectives on the origins of deviance

Early studies of social deviance, especially studies of criminality, often sought a psychological explanation for what was essentially **socially abnormal** behaviour. Behaviour seen as socially unacceptable was assumed to be caused by a defective personality or a certain physiological type or, in more sophisticated views, as arising out of a breakdown of the normal controls over innate human tendencies to follow 'base' instincts and passions.

Organicist functionalist theories viewed society as a normally healthy organism. Social deviance was seen by analogy as an 'illness' or malfunction which must be treated and cured by society. In this **social pathological** approach people exhibiting problem behaviour were seen as 'sick', dysfunctional members of society who had been inadequately socialised into accepting basic social values and who went on to violate the norms and moral expectations of society. This suggests that a normal, healthy society is harmonious and functions in an orderly manner, with a high degree of consensus between people. It leads to an assumption that the origins of deviance – the 'fault' – must lie within individuals and their groups rather than within society as a whole.

One of the problems with this view is that if a society is so well ordered, how did the deviant group, which forms part of that society, originate the deviance? Inadequate socialisation, for example, points to a flaw in the society and its socialising mechanisms rather than to the individual or group being socialised.

An alternative functionalist approach holds that deviance can be **functional for society**. Crime waves, for example, may be mechanisms for redefining the boundaries of the acceptable and the unacceptable in society. It is by controlling and punishing deviants that we can set and remind everyone of society's standards. This implies that deviance may be partly 'caused' by a desire on the part of powerful members of society to maintain control. If deviance did not exist, it might be necessary to invent it to get the rest of us to behave properly. This resembles the idea that the visibility of the symptoms of illness and disability act as a warning to the rest of us to guard our health.

The **systems functionalist** perspective sees society as a complex whole with interdependent parts which are, in normal conditions, co-ordinated. Social change becomes the main source of deviance in such a society since it creates disorder. Technological change, population movements and economic fluctuations all threaten social stability and bring about a dysjunction between the different elements of society. This theory still holds a view of society as normally harmonious and social problems or deviance as aberrations from the norm. However, social change is an inherent characteristic of most social systems. It is not abnormal; if anything, it is inevitable.

For the functionalist, consensus is treated as normal and disorganisation or change as abnormal. Functionalists will seek remedies for deviance by advocating mechanisms for coping with the rate of social change. Associated ideologies and social policies devised to resolve deviance and social problems rarely call any of society's basic forms and assumptions into question. They usually suggest ways of strengthening those agencies which exist to control deviance and say that problems can be solved by a return to the *status quo* or some mythical basic values. Such responses usually require improvements in child socialisation, formal education, legislation, the police, the judiciary and the penal system; these **agencies of social control** would be expected to perform the function already assigned to them more rigorously.

Interactionist theories hold that deviance originates in the social interaction between individuals and between and within groups, that **deviant behaviour is learned in a deviant environment**. Initially, it was argued that criminality, for example, was learned by contact with criminal groups whose values, attitudes and norms were being passed on in a socialisation process (Sutherland 1949). This notion clearly did not fit all forms of deviance: many individuals escape a deviant environment and go on to live normal lives, while some individuals become deviant without acquaintanceship with a deviant environment.

Subsequent interactionist theories concentrated on the **labelling** process. Lemert (1972) argued that individuals become deviant if they are defined or labelled as such. If society considers particular acts to be deviant, anyone doing them is defined as deviant. Once again labelling cannot explain the origins of all forms of deviance since some crimes are carried on in secret without the opportunity for societal reaction. In other words, individuals already know they are doing something deviant and do not allow others to know about it.

Interactionism concentrates on the **micro-politics** of socialisation and labelling, to the neglect of the **macro-politics** of the larger society, which frames the narrower labelling process. Furthermore, the relativism inherent in this approach suggests that the causes of deviance always lie in the wider society, while minimising the self-conscious control of individuals over their own behaviour. It becomes harder to blame anyone for their deviance. For example, the remedy for deviance suggested by this perspective might lie in us all having increased tolerance of problematic behaviour.

The **conflict perspective** sees society as composed of groups with opposing interests and values in competition with one another and/or in direct conflict over those interests. Deviance arises out of this conflict, and the nature of the conflict influences which group's point of view is taken in defining deviance. For example, militant trade unionism is seen as a social problem by capitalists, whereas capitalism and undemocratic managerial power are seen as a problem by trade unionists. For a capitalist employer strikes are a form of social deviance. For a unionist a tyrannical manager is displaying problematic behaviour. 'Property is theft' for someone who thinks it unjust for those who already have a great deal of wealth to use it to acquire more at the expense of those who own little. Marxist criminals could justify burglary on the grounds that they have merely found another way of appropriating property.

Owing to the variety of conflict theories, the remedies or solutions also vary widely: from attempts to achieve consensus and resolve disputes, through collective bargaining, to the inevitability of a revolution which might remove the basis for conflicts of interests. One problem with conflict theory explanations of deviance relates to the degree to which the groups involved self-consciously recognise their opposing interests and values. Complex **mechanisms of ideology formation** have to be used to account for why certain groups do not recognise their 'true' interests and instead adopt the values of the groups to which they should stand opposed.

Smoking offers an example. Why do those who are most deprived in society continue to engage in a habit which will damage their own health and the health of their families and friends, will reduce their life chances and will shorten their life span? They pay, for the privilege of doing this, money which will go into the pockets of a group of wealthy people – investors in and owners of tobacco companies – who use that money to improve their own life and health chances.

Exercise

As we discussed in earlier chapters, theories, ideologies and the policies which they generate are often buried in popular perspectives on problems. Find some recent newspaper, television or radio commentaries on selected accounts of some deviant act or socially problematic issue or event. Draw out the implicit theoretical perspective(s) being adopted by the commentators.

Do the same to the accounts of healthy and unhealthy practices you considered in the exercises in the Chapter 11.

Following a deviant career

One of the best ways of understanding social deviance is to trace the stages of reaction that individuals may experience once they commit abnormal acts. At each stage we can consider the various social processes that may influence how a **deviant career** progresses. The career concept draws on interactionist perspectives and was first applied by Thomas Scheff (1966) to mental illness. By stepping through a flow chart (Figure 12.1) we can focus attention on critical incidents in a person's life and the alternative biographical pathways that could occur depending on the social reactions to their behaviour.

This approach helps to demonstrate how behaviour as diverse as crime, delinquency, homosexuality, mental illness, disability and physical illness can be subject to similar social processes and produce similar responses in individuals and groups.

Starting at step (1) in Figure 12.1 we can imagine individuals behaving 'normally'. Without lengthy debate about what is meant by 'normal' treat this as an assumption that people are engaging in their usual social behaviour and activities, break no rules and give no cause for complaint from their usual associates. Then, for some reason or a whole variety of diverse causes (2), they behave in a way in which they have not behaved before (3). They might break some rules of courtesy, commit violence, steal from a department store or break out in perspiration and faint.

The vague and imprecise nature of many of society's rules means that whether or not any rules are deemed to have been broken is open to question. Many rules are **tacit social norms** about what counts as proper behaviour. Such norms are conveyed and reinforced in everyday social encounters. Other rules are regarded as important enough to require their being written down and enacted in law. The extent to which deviant behaviour will be regarded as 'rule-breaking' behaviour will depend on a variety of factors, the most important of which are listed in the box at stage (3) and discussed in detail below.

Determinants of 'rule-breaking'

(a) The **degree**, the **amount** and the **visibility** of the rule-breaking behaviour refers to objective features of the deviant act itself. How extensive is the damage done? Activities vary in the degree and frequency with which they break rules. Fainting briefly once is not such a problem as being unconscious for hours or fainting frequently. Deviant activities can also vary in their visibility. Someone suffering from a mild neurosis is less likely to attract attention than is someone who thinks they are Napoleon and dresses accordingly.

Visibility may be particularly enhanced by the publication of statistics. Official health statistics allow us to see the objective increase in the range and types of illness, but the social reality of illness only becomes noticeable, requiring action, when the statistics are collected and published. If isolated individuals suffer the effects of illness in silence, the extent of the problem is difficult for the rest of us to see.

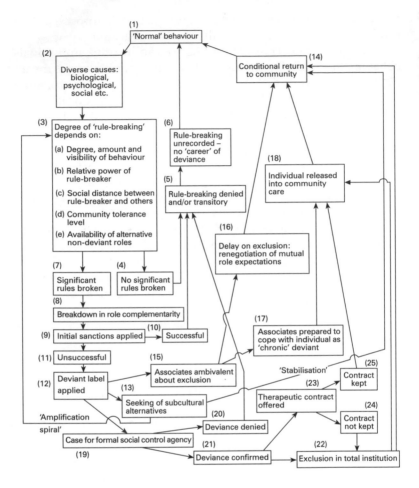

Figure 12.1   Flow chart of processes involved in 'deviant career' (based on charts by W. Buckley and T. Scheff as reported in Scheff 1966)

(b) The **power** of the rule-breakers relative to their associates and to the rest of the community also affects the way in which they will view the rule-breaking behaviour. For example, Adolf Hitler had sufficient authority to maintain the support of many German people while breaking rules about the sanctity of human life, which permitted Jewish persecution. Hitler's authority was a combination of charisma and the legal/rational authority (see Chapter 2) of distinguished scientists, psychiatrists and medical practitioners whose eugenicist perspectives were used to endorse inhuman behaviour. The power of the rule-breakers relative to the rest of the population could be such that the rule-breakers could convince observers that the rules being broken were unimportant, did not apply to them or ought to be contravened.

(c) The **social distance** between the people who break the rules and those viewing the deviant activity also matters. This is related to 'power' but refers to the social proximity of the rule-breakers and other social groups. An example here might be when you see a friend's or neighbour's children misbehaving. It is difficult to admonish the children as severely as if you had been their parent. There is more social distance between you and the children, as acquaintances, than between the parent and the children as members of the same household. One of the major difficulties of controlling deviant groups is their separation from the rest of society. People with disabilities who do not mix with the larger society are maximising their social distance and, in so doing, may minimise the possibility of being penalised by the intolerant.

(d) Communities or social groups will vary in their tolerance for different kinds of rule-breaking depending on the values they hold. How bothered are people about seeing homeless people and beggars, in various states of physical discomfort, on the street? Is this seen as a necessary consequence of policies discouraging health and welfare dependency cultures? Or is the community so concerned that law enforcement agencies have to 'clean up' the environment?

The idea of a **community tolerance level** emphasises the importance of understanding the socio-cultural context in which deviant acts occur. It is possible that the deviant and normal perspectives may coincide. Deviants may acknowledge their actions as wrongful but be unable to help themselves, such as if they show compulsive sexual misbehaviour over which they feel they have no control. Or they might justify their actions from their peculiar socio-cultural circumstances, such as stealing when poor and excusing the theft as necessary to avoid starvation.

However, deviant and community perspectives may contradict each other, so that deviants intentionally contravene community rules. Clarifying deviants' intent and their attitude to communal values is vital when assessing guilt and deciding on punishment. Even the most serious crimes can be subject to less severe punishment if rule-breakers are able to show that they acted unintentionally. Premenstrual syndrome (PMS) has been offered as a defence and justification for leniency for wives who murder their husbands. The rule-breakers' power relative to others is again important here as the system of values in any society is not equally determined by all members of society: some people are more concerned than others to generate dominant social values or are more able to effect changes in them or reinforce them. Thus PMS has to be diagnosed by medical practitioners for it to stand as an acceptable defence.

(e) Finally, the degree to which others view an act as rule-breaking depends on the **availability of alternative non-deviant roles**. This depends upon rule-breakers convincing others that what is going on is, in fact, either normal or not wrongful behaviour. Drug addicts or alcoholics may try to disguise the symptoms of their addiction by feigning an alternative, less morally judged, temporary illness.

The extent to which behaviour is regarded as breaking significant rules will depend on a combination of these variables (a to e). For example, the community tolerance level, the lack of power of others to detect, the lack of visibility and so on may be such that, in most cases, the act of exceeding the speed limit to a minor degree, where it is not generally considered dangerous to do so, would be condoned by many people. Similarly, minor thefts of equipment from one's workplace can be regarded as an occupational 'perk'. Both are, strictly, illegal acts but may not be viewed as serious.

Exercise

Take a range of examples of different types of crime, illness and disability and compare them with regard to these criteria. You might care to do this with experience of deviant acts of your own! How did you behave and how did these criteria affect others' judgements about whether serious rule-breaking took place?

Subject to all these criteria, observers of the deviant act will assess whether or not significant rules have been broken. If no significant rules have been broken or if there is general agreement that the rules are inappropriate (4), the rule-breaking will be denied or regarded as transitory (5), the deviant activity will go unrecorded (6) and the rule-breakers will not be defined as criminal, ill or insane.

Since the deviant activity has not been regarded as serious rule-breaking, the deviants might continue to behave in this manner (3) until the activity occurs so frequently that it comes to be regarded as 'normal' behaviour. Changes in language use provide examples of this in the form of the growing tolerance of swearing or blaspheming in public. Alternatively, the deviants themselves might recognise their behaviour as breaking some minor rules and may decide no longer to continue breaking them, reverting to normal behaviour (1).

When serious rule-breaking occurs (7) individuals will have failed to sustain an acceptable role performance. They have caused a breakdown in **role complementarity** (8). You will remember from Chapter 3 that this refers to how mutual expectations of future behaviour are built up through social interactions over time. As long as mutual expectations complement each other we can all perform our social roles harmoniously. If established rules are broken, our expectations of each other will no longer match, and we will find it difficult to orient our behaviour with respect to one another. We may no longer be able to predict confidently how others might behave in a given situation; they might break rules which could offend, threaten or injure us, and the simple trust which is the essence of social order will have broken down.

People who break the rules to this extent will find initial **sanctions** being applied to them (9), which attempt to get them to behave normally again. Sanctions can vary widely in extremity. For example, someone who goes into a catatonic trance (a condition in which the suffering individual will appear to have no awareness of the surrounding environment) will show no response to sensory stimuli and will not hear or see anyone. People have been known to try every device from calm talk, to shouting at, to even violently beating the individual into responding. Sanctions of a more subtle kind can be applied by demeanour and vocal intonation even in an everyday conversation. Think of how you recognise the kind of situation in which you might receive laughter in response to telling a dirty joke and those situations in which you judge the joke would be frowned upon.

The nature and success of these sanctions will again vary according to the variables listed in box (3). In addition, the deviants' attitudes to those applying the sanctions and their values are vital. Initial sanctions are more likely to succeed and less likely to be extreme if the deviance is not excessive, others are more powerful than the deviants and not too socially distant from them, where the values transgressed are not too serious, where there are no alternative non-deviant roles and where the deviants essentially agree that they have broken some rules which ought to be kept. It is in this way that health care professionals can induce patients to play the sick role 'properly': not to complain too much, not to make too many demands on precious time, not to ask too many awkward questions. Stockwell (1973) has pointed out how deviation from an acceptable sick role will call forth sanctions from professional carers.

If sanctions are successful, rule-breaking behaviour can be treated as a temporary aberration (10). The aberration may be unrecorded and the individuals will not be characterised as being 'deviant' or 'ill' (5 and 6). Thereafter, the individuals can return to a condition of 'normal' behaviour (1) to demonstrate that they are, after all, worthy members of society.

Deviant behaviour kept to this level is known as **primary deviation**. It depends upon the willingness and ability of the deviants to obey the sanctions applied to their behaviour. If the sanctions applied are unsuccessful (11), however, and the individuals continue with their rule-breaking behaviour, they will be regarded as more permanently deviant and defined by their associates as 'criminal', 'ill' or 'insane' (12). It is with the application of such **labels** that the process of **secondary deviation** begins. Labels are a means of attaching acts to people. If others begin to think of and react to individuals as 'criminal' or 'insane', since we get most of our ideas about ourselves from interaction with others, these individuals will come to see themselves as criminal or insane.

Labelling

The **labelling** concept views deviance not as a characteristic of the actual behaviour but as defined by the societal reaction to that behaviour. Labelling an individual or act as problematic sets in motion a process of action and reaction which accentuates departures from the norm. Individuals become deviant if defined as such. Communities use labels so that they know how to deal with rule-breakers and what kind of behaviour to expect from them. It is a way of re-establishing some form of role complementarity.

One consequence is that the traits of deviance are seen as governing most aspects of the deviant's life. People find it hard to believe that criminals can have a moral code. It is assumed that if individuals can transgress *some* rules and values, they can contravene *all* rules and values. Similarly, once the label 'homosexual' has been assigned to individuals, behaviour previously regarded as neutral may be re-examined for evidence of homosexual traits suggested by popular stereotypes. People with a noticeable disability may be seen as disabled in all aspects of their lives and therefore helpless, unable to communicate or take decisions about their own lives. As Rose and Platzer (1993) point out even professional carers have to examine their own prejudices.

Another consequence is that it may encourage labelled individuals to identify more strongly with any group in which their behaviour is less likely to be considered 'sick', 'abnormal' or 'wrong' (13). A closer integration with a group with which they can identify might be done out of a sense of injustice; they may feel that they have been unfairly maligned. Alternatively, membership of a **deviant subculture** might be specifically sought in order more easily to engage in deviant activity. People suffering from an illness or disability may feel more comfortable in the company of others with a common complaint.

Secondary deviation can lead to a fundamental reorganisation of attitudes, roles and, possibly, one's self-concept. In this way deviants can become what other people believe them to be. They can acquire from the group a developed set of motives which can be employed to justify, rationalise or legitimise their deviant behaviour. Homosexuals have learned the vocabulary of **resistance to medicalisation** in the company of other homosexuals (Weeks 1981).

Stigmatisation

When labelling is denigratory we **stigmatise** the individual. In some societies this marking of deviants is physical. In medieval times lepers wore bells to warn people of their approach. Some Muslim fundamentalist societies will cut off the hands, feet or limbs of people according to the severity of their crimes, thereby leaving a permanent, visible mark of their guilt. In other societies the marking can be done with a word or a name. In more bureaucratic societies the marking is done with documents – such as criminal records or case notes.

The consequences of bearing a stigma was first analysed in detail by Goffman (1968a). He pointed out that we apply negative labels to people when they are not behaving as we expect. His main concern is with how the visibility of the stigma can be controlled in order to **manage a 'spoiled' identity**. Stigmatised people adopt strategies for either revealing or concealing their deviance in order to manage how others perceive them.

People with grand mal epilepsy, for example, have to choose between whether to warn people to expect a convulsion and how to cope with it, and simply hoping that they will not have attacks in public. One of the reasons epilepsy has been stigmatised is due to its unpredictability, and even 'minor' forms of epilepsy can have major identity management consequences (Iphofen 1990). Someone in a wheelchair, however, has little choice about revealing their handicap. What they have to manage is other people's assumptions about what they are capable of doing physically and mentally.

Tragically, even the terminally ill can be stigmatised by the public knowledge of their imminent death. Relatives and carers can go to so much trouble to avoid talk of death that the situation can become socially stressful. In effect a dying person may be treated as socially deviant and handled carefully to avoid emotional difficulties and embarrassment. Even the dying person might try to manage their identity and avoid discussion of topics which they sense that others cannot handle.

Stigmatised people do tend to become highly **situation conscious** and quite skilled at strategies for revealing or concealing information about themselves. They might try to draw people's attention away from their stigma, disidentify with it or pass it off as something else. Some groups will be allowed to share information about their condition, while others may be excluded. Their identity may even appear fluid and fragile since they are constantly aware of having to control it.

Exercise

Is there anything about yourself that you would rather certain others did not know?

Do you have an aspect of behaviour, attitude or physical condition which you believe others might stigmatise?

Why did you initially hide the information?

Why did you decide to disclose it (if you did)?

Why have you carried on hiding the information (if you have)?

How do you go about controlling information about it? What do you say or do to manage your identity and prevent it from becoming 'spoiled'?

Have you observed this phenomenon in others? What techniques have you seen them use or do you suspect that they use?

Deviancy amplification

At this stage (13) a process of **deviancy amplification** might occur. This model for societal reactions to deviance was initially developed by Leslie Wilkins (1965). He suggested that labelling and stigmatisation leads to the **isolation and alienation** of deviants from society. Barred from participation in normal society and culture, deviants may feel resentful and hostile, reject social standards and seek status and comradeship among others like themselves. This creates an opportunity for an increase in deviant behaviour. There is a further reaction by society to what it sees as an increasing threat. Stricter measures are taken against the deviants, who then feel further resentment, identify even more closely with the deviant group and further increase their deviance, and so the spiral goes on. Once segregated, both society and the deviant group suffer from a lack of information about each other, thereby accentuating their separation (Cohen 1971).

In the modern world the mass media are the means whereby the deviant and society gain most of their information about each other. The media are instrumental in making people aware of behaviour which is potentially deviant by acting as **moral entrepreneurs**. They assume a right to set societal attitudes to events and people tend to accept these attitudes as representative of the general societal attitude. The media keep the whole process of action and reaction between deviant and society in the public eye.

The mass media obviously cannot report everything that happens in the world, so they select items for reportage according to their **newsworthiness**. This produces a distorted view of society. Ordinary, everyday events are not news; the reporter seeks out unusual or sensational events and exaggerates them for journalistic effect, which means that they are shown on their worst side, with public fears and moral indignation being emphasised in order to create a **moral panic**.

This happens because of the competitive structure of mass communications. Newspapers compete against newspapers and against radio and television for their audience. The public want interesting information, which means that they would rather hear about sensational events than ordinary ones. In order to retain their audiences the media have to **sensationalise** real events. Threats from BSE, *E. coli*, salmonella, 'killer bugs' and so on make good news when presented as plagues or epidemics. The moral irresponsibility of those who 'cause' the spread, either as carriers or ineffective bureaucrats, is easily cultivated. Initial panic reactions to HIV and AIDS patients offer a forceful example.

The amplification process is intensified by the segregated situation of social control agents. Medical practitioners, for example, lead lives separated from much of the community since they work long and unusual hours. Just as the police have more to do with criminals than with law-abiding citizens, so health care professionals have more to do with ill than with healthy people. Mutual isolation leads to reliance on partial media accounts.

Amplification does not apply to all kinds of deviance, and an amplification spiral cannot go on indefinitely. The level of deviance tends to stabilise and even decrease after a time. It may be that the number of deviants becomes so great that they can no longer be regarded as deviants. Think of how unusual very long hair on men or boys was considered to be just over three decades ago. This deviance became commonplace and is now barely worthy of comment. Another possibility is that the deviants are eliminated from society. The Pilgrim Fathers, deviants from dominant English religion, emigrated to North America and set up their own society in isolation from the old. Yet another possibility is a change in cultural values due to communication. If the deviants and society find a channel of communication, either or both may be changed. Thus homosexuals are now less likely to be seen as deviants after legal and moral reforms within society, although the moral panic surrounding early AIDS cases could have started the amplification spiral off again.

The mass media themselves, catalysts for the original amplification of deviance, may also be factors in its diminution. As time passes the particular topic in question, purely through continuous exposure, is no longer newsworthy and is gradually dropped, thus removing it from the public eye.

Exercise

Take an example of recent reporting of an epidemic, viral outbreak or growth of incidence of a particular condition.

Look at the range of media treatments of this one topic.

Look at how health care professionals' and health bureaucrats' comments are reported.

Look at editorial comment within newspapers.

See what evidence there is for amplification, how it happened and whether it stabilised.

Deviant subculture

Having found a suitable subculture (13) it is feasible that individuals can be permitted a conditional return to the community (14). For example, homosexuals may be allowed their deviance if they confine their deviant behaviour to those social spheres where it is accepted, but only on condition that they do not draw attention to it in predominantly heterosexual spheres. From there a *new* kind of 'normal' behaviour can be established.

Another opportunity for a conditional return to the community can arise if people do not want to pass the deviants on to a formal social control agency (15). Associates may delay excluding deviant individuals and give them an opportunity to renegotiate their mutual role expectations (16). Clearly, this conditional return to the community (14) does not involve behaving in the same way as one behaved before; this behaviour will be based on the new sets of expectations that people will have of each other.

Alternatively, associates may view the individuals as 'chronic' deviants and decide that they will deal with them as such (17). In the case of mental illness, for example, this may involve individuals being cared for by their families or, in addition, paying regular visits to day centres (18). Their return to the community would then be conditional upon their acceptance of community care for chronic 'invalids'. Once again, a new kind of normal behaviour would be established which allows for the changes in the regular activities of the individuals brought about by their 'illness'.

Agencies of social control

Once labelled, attempts will be made to control or cure deviants by various formal agencies (19). The first of such **social control agents** might be a doctor, a social worker, a policeman or a nurse. If rule-breakers are apprehended in the act of rule-breaking, police intervention might be automatic. In other cases associates might be aware of deviants' behaviour and others might not, so that the associates have actively to seek the assistance of a formal social control agency. Think of the parents of a growing child with disabilities whose care as a baby is less physically and psychologically demanding. As the child grows the parents may have no alternative but to seek the assistance of some formal care agency.

The social control agency also has two alternatives open to it. It could fail to confirm the deviant status of individuals (20). That is, it can deny that individuals are as ill, as bad or as mad as others say they are. In the case of criminal acts the police might deny deviancy on the grounds that there is insufficient evidence on which to base a charge. In the case of mental illness a diagnosing primary care physician might be influenced by the degree of illness as against a perception of the shortage of hospital places for mental patients. For whatever reason, if this does happen, individuals can move to the stage where rule-breaking is either denied, regarded as insignificant or transitory (5). No career of deviance would then be officially recorded (6) and individuals could return to normal existence within the community. Of course, if individuals continue to break rules, others can continue to present them to the social control agency until it is finally forced to confirm deviant status (21).

Once deviant status is officially confirmed, another series of alternatives opens up. Both of these depend on how chronic the rule-breaking is seen to be. If it is viewed as serious, the authorities will ensure that the individuals are cared for in a **total institution** (22) such as an asylum or a prison, entry to and departure from which is tightly regulated (Goffman 1968b). At this stage individuals have been clearly identified as severe rule-breakers.

After a specified or indefinite time in a total institution individuals may be released into the community again – (18) and/or (14) – and adopt a form of normal behaviour (1), but a form which usually takes into account their institutional experience. The social stigma of having been in an institution might never be lost. The initial deviant label of 'mental patient', for example, will now be replaced by 'ex-mental patient', and the behaviour of the deviant individuals' associates may be adjusted accordingly.

Excluding deviants in a total institution is a last resort. Once deviance is confirmed (21) it may been possible to offer individuals a **therapeutic contract** (23). This means that individuals can be put on probation or asked regularly to attend a psychiatrist or therapy group. In this case responsibility is placed on the deviant individuals to make a conscious choice which will affect how they are subsequently to be treated. If they fail to keep the contract (24), the authorities would be justified in affirming the chronicity of their rule-breaking and confining them to a total institution (22). However, if individuals do manage to keep to the therapeutic contract (25), they could be judged as to some degree 'stable' or will at least be considered conditionally capable of a return to conventional roles and conventional behaviour, moving from (18) to (14) to (1).

Exercise

Apply this flow chart to various health- and illness-related activities. Look at smoking tobacco, using illegal drugs, drinking alcohol, physical disability, mental disability, being ill with AIDS, body scarring through accident, tattooing and body piercing.

Apply the chart to incidents which you have personally experienced. Was there a time when a critical event and people's reactions to you moved you through these stages?

Or have you seen this happen to someone else – a friend, an associate or a client?

Critical influences include changes in the community tolerance level over time and the role of control agencies. Make use of your understanding of power and authority and of role relationships established in earlier exercises. Compare the key stages of different illness events.

Conclusion

Using this notion of a deviant career we see how a variety of possible alternative paths open up for individuals who become involved in deviant acts. It shows the importance of societal reactions to deviance and the deviant individuals' responses to those reactions in determining their fate. From this viewpoint no form of human behaviour can be seen as inherently deviant in itself. What makes it deviant is the attitude of society and its agents toward that behaviour.

Many kinds of behaviour regarded as deviant in our society have, at other times and in other societies, been regarded as normal. Drug-taking, prostitution and sex with children all provide examples of such behaviour. Social deviance and social problems arise when society's tolerance level is surpassed and some ordered, systematic action for the correction or elimination of the deviant behaviour is deemed necessary.

When health care professionals participate in social control they may be balancing a concern for public health and safety with the personal interests of a client. To label something as an illness deprives the individual of the opportunity to plead rational intent and argue for a change in attitudes toward and tolerance of the behaviour exhibited. Zola (1972) showed how calling something an illness both depoliticises the condition and disempowers the 'sufferer'. Drug use could be seen as a way of life or a leisure pursuit were it not for the fact that society will not tolerate it. Health care professionals who are complicit in medicalising the condition treat such a way of life as addiction and seek a cure, thereby maintaining without challenge the boundaries of acceptability in society. Once again power and inequality lie at the root of understanding health- and illness-related behaviours.

In the next chapter we put together many of the concepts we have introduced to you in order to question the stereotypical views held about some fundamental aspects of contemporary life:

work in the home, unemployment, leisure and recreation and some ideas about the human body.

Further reading

Pearson, G. (1975) *The Deviant Imagination*, London: Macmillan.
Prins, H. (1995) *Offenders, Deviants or Patients?* (2nd edn), London: Routledge.
Of the many introductory books on social deviance these are the best for health care professionals. They are comprehensive, sensitive and insightful, with appropriate case study illustrations.

Chapter 13 The Costs of 'Free' Time

Formal and informal divisions of labour can radically shape opportunities for the use of time and the types of leisure which are available to different groups. Leisure entails a set of activities clearly different from the world of work, yet 'free' time is much harder to find than we suppose. Clarifying who does or does not have leisure is particularly important for understanding who is 'available' to support health care in the home or who has easy access to healthy leisure activities.

Non-employed work

As we discussed in Chapter 6 it may be difficult to recognise or acknowledge some kinds of tasks as being 'real work' and, in consequence, they may be confused with leisure. One example of this is housework. Housework-related activities may include those seen as care work, including the kinds of care that maintain or restore health or alleviate illness.

Exercise

What sort of work is entailed in domestic/household tasks?

The following are a list of tasks which most people have to do. In your household, who does them, how often do they have to be done and how are they viewed? Conduct an audit of who does what and ask why.

cont'd

Task	Who?	Alienating? (which dimension?)	Satisfying?	Frequency?
Grocery shopping				
Clothes shopping				
Durables shopping				
Clothes washing				
Ironing				
Preparing meals				
Cooking				
Dishwashing				
Vacuuming				
Washing floors				
Dusting				
Cleaning bathrooms				
Cleaning toilets				
Tidying				
Gardening				
Motor repairs				
Personal hygiene of the young...				
... the ill... or...				
... the old... or				
... the disabled				
Decorating				
DIY				

There is often clear **gender variation in household tasks**. Those which entail caring for others tend to be conducted by females. The more regularly repetitive tasks which we call housework are often done by women but are not seen as work. Work at home is invisible work and is unpaid, so it is not taken as seriously. The assumption is made that it is done during unregulated free time, so is unstructured. There is little doubt, however, that it is laborious, repetitive, time-consuming and monotonous but still requires knowledge and considerable organising skills, and entails many responsibilities in terms of the needs of the members of the household. As a consequence it can be just as stressful as formal, paid employment and even more relentless. Its contribution to the economic structure may be trivialised, thereby disempowering women, who are more often responsible for undertaking such work.

It may be less obvious whether household repairs or DIY count as housework. In thinking about why this is consider whether particular repairs or DIY jobs have to be done every week and which gender is usually seen as responsible for them. Readily identifiable one-off tasks may seem less trivial and can therefore be more readily made visible.

Responsibility for housework becomes a double burden on women with employed work responsibilities. It is work activity which brings no guaranteed income, although its social and economic value is beginning to be acknowledged in modern divorce settlements and divisions of property of cohabiting couples who separate. Because it is trivialised it brings responsibilities without power.

Oakley's (1974) work has shown how the allocation of household tasks and the resources for doing them is based on processes of informal agreement within households or families. This, too, is likely to be based on an unequal domestic order. Men are more likely to control the family purse. Where men are the main earners in families and where households are poorer, they are less likely to hand over an adequate share of money for housekeeping. They are more likely to keep aside a larger personal share for small treats such as cigarettes. Graham's (1984) research on poorer families reveals that women are most likely to go without food and personal needs to supply the rest of the household with basics such as food and fuel.

Household tasks have traditionally been divided along male/female lines. The more egalitarian symmetrical partnerships between spouses anticipated by Young and Wilmott (1975) has not occurred as expected. Detailed work carried out in the 1980s on household work and incomes has indicated that such arrangements are more common in younger middle-class households. Undesirable household tasks are most likely to be allocated according to the relative power of particular family members. There is more likely to be task-sharing and more clearly recognised leisure time for women in households where women have paid jobs and more bargaining power (Deem 1986). Otherwise, it is most likely to be female members of the household who assume the bulk of such household tasks.

This has important implications for health professionals' assumptions about who will and who should take over 'caring' roles within families (Finch 1989). It may be taken for granted that female partners or relatives may be able and willing to undertake such roles. Given current patterns of women's paid and unpaid work, they are less likely than men to be able to draw on adequate resources (income, contacts, benefits or equipment) to support such work. If their lives are already subject to less well-structured and conflicting demands, care work may not be easily undertaken. If the work includes tasks which reflect housework or domestic responsibilities, this may have consequences for how much formal status and value, including economic value, is given to their own work. (Compare this with disputes between health professionals about who is responsible for tidying the workplace.) In any case the emotional costs of caring are often ignored or played down. Emotional labour is demanding in both a physical and a psychological sense (James 1989; Smith 1992).

Unemployment

Such debate underlines the problematic effects on a person's social status if they are not engaged in some form of paid employment. They also call into question any notion that unemployment is an easy lifestyle option likely to be freely chosen by most unemployed people. Since status and identity come from being in an occupation, a profession or a position within an organisation, **unemployment stigmatises** in that it entails loss of status, power and self-esteem. For people who have grown accustomed to work which gives a routine structure and focus to the day, not working can appear to be aimless and alienating.

Because employment is a major source of income, unemployment remains the greatest single cause of poverty. Loss of independent income means a loss of financial privileges and the resources for maintaining living standards for all dependent members of the household. Greater proportions of income have to be spent on necessities, so unemployment gives rise to **enforced leisure** without the means to appreciate it to the full. This can lead to **social isolation**. Social relationships cost money. Eating meals at home or out, buying a round of drinks and many leisure activities cannot be sustained with friends who still have enough money. Since mixing with other unemployed people becomes more likely, on-the-job contacts which may have given rise to further work are often lost. Professionals facing unemployment for the first time can find the experience particularly traumatic. House repossessions and being unable to afford customary entertainments or family holidays abroad can underline the fragility of their lifestyle.

The unemployed are often accused of maintaining an alternative **black economy** of unofficial trading and service provision. However, 'fiddles' are dependent on being in employment since they are difficult to sustain without an infrastructure of equipment, transport, communications and contacts. Most modern societies are geared to contractual agreements and a money economy. Women are particularly disadvantaged by their reliance on their less valued personal time and labour, for example, if they do undeclared cleaning, childminding or home sewing (Poland 1992).

There are marked geographical variations in the nature of work and employment, so corresponding variations in the extent of unemployment are inevitable. Industry and commerce tend to locate according to the supply of human and material resources and access to the market for their products, so regional economies are subject to the fortunes of the trade cycle. This gives rise to pockets of disadvantage linked to the extent of unemployment. For example, until recently, there have been clear variations in the extent of unemployment between the North and the South of the UK. The so-called mid-1980s economic boom took place mainly in the south-east. Unemployment there was typically one-half or one-third of that in the North and the 'Celtic fringe'.

The global divide between the affluent North and the impoverished South is a consequence of traditional economic divisions. Systematic socio-economic constraints restrict opportunities for many groups readily to find work. It is becoming more difficult for younger people with fewer skills or work experience. Those aged over 45 also increasingly find that their age counts against them on the job market. Where affordable child care is not widely available, as in the UK, this often excludes women and single parents from employment.

Lengthy periods of unemployment effectively exclude people from the labour market. Employers become suspicious of the job seekers' diligence. Durable jobs are hard to find and to sustain if the routines of employed work cannot easily be re-established. The long-term unemployed are less likely to live in a comfortable house and have a new car or good clothes. They are more likely to have run down their assets, leaving them unable to replace or repair. Higher-income lifestyles are not sustainable over long periods of unemployment.

Exercise

The popular mass media and gossip may appear to support the image of unemployment as being an option freely chosen by particular groups. Myths about unemployment create prejudices which are difficult to overcome.

You may have particular impressions about why and how a person is employed, unemployed or working in other ways. One way to test your own stereotypes about unemployment and its effects is to ask yourself the following questions:

How much, in detail, do you really know about someone else's business?

How much do you assume?

How much do you tell people about your own income?

If you have engaged in any 'fiddles', what was the incentive and means for doing it?

How many people personally do you know who are truly long-term unemployed and have regular 'black economy' work?

If you know directly (as opposed to by hearsay) someone who receives welfare benefits or who does black economy work, how good is their standard of living?

Research findings (Morris 1985) have contradicted stereotypes about unemployment promoting a more egalitarian involvement in housework and carework. Where both partners are unemployed sharing of housework has proved to be less rather than more common. Unemployed men are often more unwilling to take on work which may be seen as further diminishing their self-esteem. Women are less likely to feel entitled to take leisure time. They are also more likely to experience the need to use their own labour to provide basic household needs through making and managing. Men and women may therefore experience different effects from unemployment because of different expectations in their working lives.

The controversy over who is genuinely unemployed can be exploited by governments who wish to 'massage' statistics in their own interests. Restrictive unemployment registration procedures help to disguise youth unemployment, age prejudices in employment practice, part-time temporary work, poverty and homelessness. Unemployment statistics are likely to exclude individuals experiencing various kinds of chronic sickness and disability as well as those receiving pensions. All of these may be disadvantaged by the experiences of unemployment detailed above but may be much less likely to be recognised as such.

Unemployment and health

Reducing unemployment remains a high priority for most of the major industrial societies in the West, owing in part to the evident health consequences of unemployment. Psychologically, the unemployed will experience **frustration** and a **sense of relative deprivation** due to unfulfilled expectations and an inability to escape structural constraints on available employment and gain full access to leisure and amenities. There will be reduced ability to meet basic needs for warmth, housing, clothing and nutrition.

Most of the indicators of anxiety and depression generated by unemployment emerge in the first three months. There may be character changes and new family tensions. Eating and behavioural disorders are common among children, and depression among spouses. Many people blame themselves for their unemployment. Their sense of guilt stops them from seeing themselves as victims of economic trends or government policy. This perception is exacerbated by 'welfare scrounger' stereotypes which are still popularly held. As a result acute mental health problems can appear.

After adjusting for the effects of social class and age, mortality and morbidity rates for the unemployed are higher than for the employed. Regional variations in economic advantage make it more likely that unemployed people live in areas which lack adequate health care, social services and transport and leisure facilities.

Professional health carers have to remain attuned to their own stereotypes about employment and unemployment and about who is appropriate or available to take on informal care tasks. It cannot be assumed that the unemployed are available for care work. They may have less time, fewer resources, less money, less social support and more stress. Women may have other invisible and stressful commitments, and it may be all too easy to impose on them and see their commitments as less important.

Recreation

Any discussion of unemployment highlights the close links between employment and leisure through social networks and social interactions. More visible forms of leisure are very clearly linked to employment by being seen as 'earned'. Such recreational forms are given a structure by the organisation of the world of employment. Recreation takes place at weekends or evenings after the 'working day' or week is over. Ironically, people who are seen as having 'proper' jobs are given more entitlement to leisure. Such jobs also provide more resources to spend on leisure. Leisure may be more problematic for many social groups with less access to full-time employment, including the unemployed, women, people with disabilities and older people, despite stereotypes of such groups being 'at leisure'.

Women's leisure activities are typically those which may be undertaken alongside domestic responsibilities or are actually part of domestic responsibilities, such as sewing, cooking or even shopping. 'Time out' for them may be often short: a stop at a super-market for a cup of coffee or a pause for a chat and a cigarette. These are very different from identifiable recreational pursuits.

It may already be difficult for some people either to take leisure or to feel entitled to take leisure. Some healthier leisure activities may be expensive in terms of time, travel and equipment. They may be controlled by social groups which may be strongly gender-, class- or age-related or to which it may be difficult to gain membership without certain levels of investment. 'Unhealthy' leisure activities (for example smoking and watching television) may be the best available in the circumstances, the only ones that can be afforded or ones which maintain much-needed social contacts.

Traditional leisure activities have been clearly linked to membership of particular social groups. Mass participatory or spectator sports such as football tend to be more associated with the working class, while individual participatory activities which may be expensive – such as yacht racing or golf – are more middle- or upper-class pastimes. Cinema may be relatively classless, but opera and theatre tends to remain the preserve of the upper classes. In gender terms men are more likely to leave the house for recreation and women more likely to stay at home. Men are more likely to go to pubs and bars or go fishing; women are more likely to go to cafes, run coffee mornings or to do home crafts. Age-related recreational activities are even more marked. Children are more likely to engage in active play, use computer games or play with dolls; young people are more likely to go to clubs or raves; older people are more likely to bowl or go to tea dances. Regional variations include the preference some communities have for choirs, for brass bands or for sport. Other activities are strongly linked with ethnic identity, such as folk music, dancing or specific kinds of craft work.

Deem's (1986) work describes how opportunities for leisure are structured by the world of work. Many forms of leisure are not free but must be resourced, often through the payment of fees and the provision of travel, equipment and clothes. She also emphasises that the right to leisure time is the object of negotiation and may depend on the kinds of work in which a person is engaged.

Formal work provides entitlement and resources for leisure time. Formal jobs structure days, weeks and years within which time for leisure is made available. Other kinds of job may lack clear boundaries and may therefore continually break into leisure time. This is typical of child care, in which responsibilities may be twenty-four hours a day and in relation to which carers may find it difficult to justify or indeed to organise uninterrupted leisure, even for a chat, let alone some more organised leisure activity such as sport.

Exercise

What sort of leisure activity is done by each member of your household?

Set out and complete the following list:

**Type of leisure
engaged in**   **Member of household**

....

....

....

.... etc.

Think about:

● how is it decided who engages in which leisure activity
● what pattern there is to it (e.g. gender, age or family status).

Is this pattern similar to those of your friends, neighbours or colleagues?

Invisible support

For a wide range of reasons people do not necessarily know much about the 'non-work' activities of neighbours and, sometimes, even of family and friends. This is in part because routine leisure activities are often supported by other people's invisible work. Such forms of support include:

● lifts or escorting to hobbies, games or evening classes;
● sports and leisure club organisation, where women often provide catering, administration and audience support;
● buying and washing uniforms and sports kit;
● self-catering holidays, which often mean continuing household work, usually with fewer household aids and less local shopping knowledge to accomplish such work;

- knitting or cooking – which may be seen as hobbies or as providing for household needs.

Women's leisure is therefore not only less common, but also less visible. This is because it often has to be fitted in with other people's activities or fitted in with other duties such as shopping.

Key questions

In your list above did you include attending and being involved in church activities, visiting relatives, chatting and shopping?

Do you see these activities as work or leisure?

Your view on visiting relatives may be influenced by the expenditure of money, time and energy involved. Think of transport, tasks undertaken before or during the visits and who provides food. Perceptions may also be influenced by the relative ages and disabilities of those visited. When may it be readily assumed that a visit is 'duty' or 'a favour' rather than just for pleasure?

Whether you define shopping as work or leisure will depend on who is doing it, for what items and in what circumstances. The commercial organisation of shopping to encourage mass participation has blurred the perception of shopping as work by the provision of leisure props for shopping. Within department stores or in shopping malls there are cafes, music, street entertainments, plants and landscaping. It is an activity that may be carried out with friends or family. It is seen as a form of consumption in itself, a chance for indulgence through spending on luxury or entertainment items (O'Brien and Harris 1991).

A cost–benefit analysis of fun

Exercise

List all your leisure activities – the things you do in your spare time which you do for pleasure. List what they cost you (and others) and how they might benefit you (and others).

	Costs		Benefits	
Leisure activity	**To you**	**To society**	**To you**	**To society**
....	....	....	....	....
....	....	....	....	....
....	....	....	....	....
....	....	....	....	....
.... etc.				

You might think about whether different non-work obligations create different obligations or responsibilities for different members of the family. Did you include health items as benefits in your list? Do some non-paid work and leisure activities foster health more than others? Can the costs and benefits of physical and mental health gains from leisure activities be sensibly compared?

As we discussed earlier even play is not a free activity but structured in various ways. Fun relationships in our society are difficult to sustain without a supportive network and reciprocal exchanges of goods or activities and of communication. Available forms of leisure are continually changing. It now appears that many less traditional types of leisure are not so clearly associated with particular groups. Cheap options have been made more widely available with the development of a mass leisure industry. Many of these forms of leisure have been defined as involving people in passive and privatised consumption. Examples of these include:

- listening to recorded music;
- watching sports on television;

- film and video-watching.

It can be argued that the commercialisation of leisure has emphasised passivity for the purposes of easier selling. However, developments in information technology offer possibilities for more active technology-based leisure such as:

- music recording;
- photography;
- video recording;
- computers and the Internet;
- electronic instruments.

Women and girls are often seen as less deserving of more expensive technical leisure equipment. Gender stereotyping may also suggest that they are less competent to use such equipment, that they may need more time or space to learn to use it and that technical knowledge is less appropriate to a feminine image. Women's involvement in such active leisure pursuits is more likely to be as the passive objects of such activities (as with photographic models) or as audiences for them.

Eating

Eating is an activity which may appear simply to meet biological needs. However, like most activities, how it can be performed and what it means are intimately bound up with the social contexts in which it takes place, with cultural traditions and with personal emotions. In modern societies specialist eating places and styles have developed, together with the proliferation of **consumer identities** catered for in a mass culture of **commodification**. Most things can be turned into commodities and sold. Eating is almost always identified with leisure through being undertaken in your 'own time'. The variety of settings in which it may be undertaken therefore range from the domestic, through work organisations and fast food outlets, to hotels and restaurants.

In common with many other forms of leisure the purchase, preparation and consumption of food is closely connected to traditional, ethnic and other cultural groupings and styles. Social eating and certain styles of food may be used to mark particular occasions of social significance, including life events. In all of these, as with forms of care, women and socially disadvantaged groups are most likely to be bound up with their production. Women most often undertake the purchase and preparation of food for domestic consumption.

Eating is linked to the significance of the social occasion and its value to the group with whom it is undertaken. Orbach (1978) emphasised the role of women in feeling obliged to demonstrate caring and loving through the provision of food in routine and in celebratory ways. As Bateson (1989) points out this can increase the domestic workload and become oppressive owing to cultural expectations about females needing to provide for male needs. Together with any limitations on resources for eating, such expectations constrain individual choices in relation to potential changes of diet.

Exercise

Describe some of the social issues which a health professional may have to take into account if they want to encourage an individual to make changes in their diet in the cases of:

- a young man who spends much of his evening leisure time with male friends who frequently visit pubs;

- an older, housebound man or woman who relies on home care assistants to do their food shopping;

- an unemployed mother with three small children who lives on an out-of-town housing estate;

- a married man who is employed in strenuous physical labour;

- a sales manager who eats many meals out with clients or while travelling.

Food provides a variety of cultural objects for commodification and consumption. Whether it is seen as satisfactory relates to much more than whether it is edible or inedible. Ideas of leisure in today's society bring together notions of indulgence and choices of identity, with the variety of commodities made available through the market.

Body images

In the same way people's bodies are much more than biological entities. They can also be seen as **aesthetic images** to be presented and sometimes literally **sold as cultural objects**. This can be seen most clearly in representations of the female body. Artists have long been interested in the female form and have made use of women's bodies as objects. As new art forms emerge this use of the female form has been maintained by photographers, cinematographers, videographers and computer artists. As Marina Warner (1987) documents, through the centuries these images have fulfilled aesthetic, symbolic, allegorical and erotic functions.

All such representations reflect contemporary views held about women's place in society. The late Victorians, in their portrayal of women, emphasised characteristic Victorian values which were clearly ideals of sentimentality, domesticity and moral righteousness. The early twentieth century saw the development of one of the earliest vehicles for gender stereotyping in advertising – the calendar. By the 1950s and 1960s the female body had become not only the object of the male gaze, but also an appendage to the objects being sold and thereby relatively devalued. By the 1970s society had come to tolerate ever-fewer clothes and a focus on parts of female bodies at the expense of the whole person. At this point it could be said that the distinction between advertising and pornography was obscured, culminating in the production of the 'classic' Pirelli calendars.

The objectifying of women's bodies has become routine in advertising. As we saw in Chapter 9 advertisements which fragment the body imply that a woman is just a set of body parts: tender hands, clear skin, bright eyes, white teeth, richly coloured hair, hairless shapely legs, all separate 'bits' requiring and receiving special attention.

In a seminal work Packard (1957) discussed how advertisers took a prime place in the development of sexual stereotyping as contributing to a capitalist economy. The images they produce are based on the use of market surveys and through attempting to target buying groups with a perceptible identity. In the late 1980s women's buying groups in the UK were identified and targeted to include:

- Lively Ladies (ambitious, self-assured, materialistic);
- Avant Guardian (serious newspaper, bicycle, designer boiler suit);
- Hopeful Seeker (middle-aged mum, gentle, friendly, anxious to be liked);
- New Unromantic (hard-headed, young, working, single, childless).

Advertisers face problems when they have to sell to several of their stereotypes at once. Incorporating the ambiguities may obscure their differences and appeal to none. 'Glamour' images can create anxiety for the female spectator concerning the difference between herself and the idealised image. This occurs even though there is awareness that the image is unreal and that a great deal of hidden effort goes into the production of glamour.

Advertising presents the most rigid stereotyping. In the classic beer/lager advert the tanned muscular young man, perspiring heavily after hard physical work, is yearning for a pint; it is much less likely that hot, sweaty women will be represented in this context – except in an erotic deodorant advertisement. For much of the twentieth century this ideal has generally meant being young, white, healthy and good looking. More ethnic and age diversity can now be seen but in a limited way. It could be argued that the dominant images reflect idealised dominant groups: whiteness idealises cultural imperialism; youth idealises the active and self-sufficient, healthy and good looking.

Sontag (1982) discusses how, in pornography, we see these trends taken to their fullest extent. The image of the woman's body itself becomes an object. The pornographic image stands as a saleable commodity in its own right, a clear example of a process of dehumanisation. It is not even the actual body of the female which is turned into a commodity, but a representation of that body.

Pornography seems to mirror attitudes to sexual relations within the rest of society, relations which have much to do with control, power and domination. Indeed, some male sexual fantasies entail the subordination of women. To be attractive, women have to appear childlike, younger than men, vulnerable and submissive and thus more controllable. The purchaser of pornographic material gains control over the object in fantasy. A vicarious mastery is achieved in the act of 'gazing'. Sadistic images take the theme of mastery even further. A key media issue is often raised in this connection: the likelihood of the gazer trying to convert fantasy into fact. Thus there is much debate about the link between pornography and violent sexual crimes. Also, it is now acknowledged that one of the disadvantages of the highly publicised permissive sexual revolution of the 1960s and early 1970s was to impose demands on sexual performance, sexual behaviour and bodily performance which not everyone could live up to.

Aspects of such demands can be seen in the development of clothes fashions and bodily disciplines to alter or emphasise particular body shapes. Over the centuries both male and female groups have used corsets to achieve tight waists. Russian and Prussian soldiers in the nineteenth century wore military corsets, while Victorian women aimed for 15 inch waists. The women of a tribe in Burma successively fit copper coils to their necks in order to lengthen them. The longest neck supported in this way was 40 cm. Brassieres were developed and modified to suit contemporary preferences for female breast shapes. Practices such as these have been linked to a range of physical symptoms and illnesses which are clearly seen as secondary to the need to display culturally dominant identities.

The market offers many possible routes for personal presentation and transformation through consumption. However, it also helps to create enormous pressures on non-dominant groups to undertake such transformations. In Japan it is seen as women's responsibility to turn out well-dressed, well-ironed, clean and tidy husbands and children. The accusation of scruffiness – 'darashi ga nai' – against children or a husband involves a serious loss of face for the mother/wife. Hence the Japanese are always impeccably dressed even when in casual clothes.

The experience of such pressures, attempts to respond to them and the experience of some of these transformations can all bring their own health risks and problems. Some of these risks and problems affect individuals, while some forms of recreation may be seen as potentially risky for the wider society. These include football hooliganism and drug-taking.

Exercise

Illnesses and surgery may have social as well as physiological consequences. List some of the consequences in terms of individuals' participation in activities which could be classified as 'leisure' or 'consumption' in the following cases:

- a woman who has had a mastectomy;

- an adolescent youth with acne;

- a girl who has a growth disorder leading to her being over 6 feet tall;

- an adult man who has vitiligo (loss of skin pigmentation);

- a fifty-year-old man who has had a colostomy;

- an older woman who has had facial cosmetic surgery.

Which social consequences do you think might be seen as desirable or undesirable in terms of individuals' construction of their identities and why?

Bodies and food

Putting attitudes to food, eating and body imagery together produces major health concerns for women: **anorexia nervosa** and **bulimia**. Eating disorders in which people choose not to eat at all, to eat so little as to threaten their health and to eat excessively followed by rigorous body purges seem to be more common among young women in advanced societies. First diagnosed in the mid-nineteenth century, they have grown more common in the past twenty years but still only affect approximately 1 per cent of the female population in the West.

Among other writers Brown and Jasper (1993) relate these conditions to attempts to attain the idealised female body images portrayed by the mass media, together with the complex emotional responses to women's role in the use and preparation of food. Contemporary idealised imagery typically represents females as thinner than average (Wolf 1991). At other times, and in other societies, fatness has been idealised. Indeed, in impoverished societies women who are over average weight are taken to signify a wealthy household.

Conclusion

Understanding about different kinds of work can tell us about the pressures of undertaking 'non-work', being unemployed and taking leisure. If recreational opportunities are highly structured and legitimised by employed work roles, leisure will be notably different for different sexes and disability groups. This is relevant in considering the potential for self-care in a mass consumption society and the topic of inclusions and exclusions from health-supporting, social-networking activities.

There are many implications of this for health education, health promotion or health care. Unemployed households may have less time, fewer resources, less money and less social support available to themselves to sustain caring tasks. They may be subject to more stress. Women may have invisible and stressful multiple commitments to a range of relationships and households, and domestic tasks. It is too easy to see these commitments as less important. Certain social groups – the unemployed, women and older people – may already find it difficult to take leisure or feel entitled to take leisure, or are subjected to contradictory pressures over those things which are seen by most people as recreational. Allocating long-term care work responsibilities may reduce already limited leisure opportunities, which may, in turn, affect a household's resources for offering care.

Not all aspects of health and social care can be easily commodified or left to remain invisible. Governments feel some responsibility for certain amounts of national welfare. In the penultimate chapter we address issues associated with the distribution of power, health and caring service provision throughout society.

Further reading

Appadurai, A. (ed.) (1986) *The Social Life of Things – Commodities in Cultural Perspective*, Cambridge: Cambridge University Press.
Barthes, R. (1982) *Empire of Signs*, New York: Hill & Wang.

The above books offer some insight into modern imagery and the commodification of most things.

Falk, P. (1994) *The Consuming Body*, London, Thousand Oaks: Sage.

Mennell, S., Murcott, A. and van Otterloo, A.H. (1992) *The Sociology of Food and Eating*, London: Sage.
These works offer an accessible overview of bodies and eating.

Northrup, C. (1995) *Women's Bodies, Women's Wisdom*, London: Piatkus.
An excellent, readable book on holistic health for women which addresses many of the topics raised in this chapter.

Chapter 14 Welfare, Ill-fare, How Fair?

State welfare systems were established when public expenditure was assumed to be an inevitable part of economic growth. By the 1980s welfare spending had come to be seen by governments globally as a burden, and new ways of funding public health and welfare services had to be considered.

Welfare policy and decision-making

Providing for the health needs of individuals in advanced societies with complicated economic and occupational structures entails maintaining a balance between the resources of individuals and those provided by other agencies, including the government.

Cousins (1987) traces how the welfare state which emerged in Britain over the twentieth century was the outcome of a particular view about political and economic development. There was a consensus that the state held responsibility to provide for the physical and educational capability of its citizens, if as many as possible were actively to contribute to the life and work of the whole society. This meant drawing on a system of tax and national insurance to provide resources through official benefits, welfare, educational and health agencies or minimum universal access to basic means of living. These include food, housing, education and health. It was expected that the government would legislate and plan for **guaranteed universal access** to some minimal kinds of resource and at least equal access to others. The state was seen as the ultimate beneficiary of this arrangement in that people would be strong and healthy enough to supply industry and commerce as well as being available for the armed forces.

The success of such an arrangement must depend upon the ability of the state to command sufficient resources to meet the demands made upon it. This depends on the overall resources in the economy, the level of demands made, general agreement on resources to be contributed, and agreement that the services supplied are appropriate to needs. Perceptions of 'what is appropriate' may differ according to who is defining 'needs', as we discussed in Chapter 7.

Welfarism relies on the ability to limit demands. More recently, many governments have used free market principles to develop a system which gives greater emphasis on private services.

Balancing problems of supply and demand

Whenever unlimited demand exists for goods and services in restricted supply, some means of limiting consumer access must be applied. The mechanisms available for limiting access can range from **rationing** (more usually applied to public services) to **free market principles** (more usually applied to private and commercial goods and services). Since health is currently highly valued, such mechanisms are equally applicable to the allocation of health resources and health care services. However, neither public nor employer organisations may see it as their responsibility to provide such goods and services.

Rationing does not necessarily offer fair access to all consumers. Given that goods or services are in short supply, allowing all people equal amounts does not ensure that those in greater need will acquire a sufficient amount of the goods or services to meet their requirements. Similarly, it allows government agents to determine categories of consumer who may be deemed to have greater need or will perceive greater benefit, and to allocate goods and services accordingly.

Since the 1970s criticisms of the post-war welfare state have suggested that this system was unlikely to provide services at a sufficient level or standard to meet demands. A global economic recession with high unemployment made it increasingly difficult to resource both the economy and any expansion of welfare services. Demographic changes pointed to greater numbers of older sick people to be maintained by a system without the proportionate numbers of younger people to fund services. The widespread development of the notion of the **consumer society** has encouraged consumers actively to assert their rights and choices. This has also fuelled middle-class dissatisfaction with the restrictions of the passive role of service recipient.

A variety of social groups were, in any case, marginal to any previous consensus. These included older people, women, ethnic groups and diverse community and environmental groups. The development of new treatments and technologies in health offered the possibility of a wider range of choices in provision. However, within a rationed system these could not be made equally accessible to clients. Government and health administrators argued that new developments could be made available within a free market system. If fewer welfare-related resources were paid to fund government provision, this would allow individuals to pay for their own preferred sources of health treatment and services.

Where a system of rationing is overseen by public services, some form of government agency makes decisions on who gets what goods and services, and how much of each they get. Within a free market system of provision, access to goods and services is determined by a contract between a purchaser and a provider. Such contracts take the form of a promise to pay a certain amount in return for specified goods. The ordinary bank note is such a contract. At times of economic hardship or crisis in a society, rationing may be introduced by a government to ensure that the bulk of the population is not deprived of minimal goods and services. If there is a perception that policies are failing to meet acceptable standards of delivery, attempts may also be made to deploy rationing, perhaps combined with market principles in what is regarded as an '**optimal mix**'. This currently applies to the system of health care in the UK.

The concept of a 'free market' is a misnomer as no market can be, in practice, truly free. A free market can only exist under the conditions that economists refer to as **perfect competition**. This is an idealised situation in which demand and supply are equally matched and where all consumers and all suppliers are fully informed about all the goods available in the market and their prices. It would then be possible for decisions about purchasing and producing to be mutually adjusted. In such a situation everyone could get what they wanted, and there would be no dissatisfied producers or consumers.

In contrast, the situation which applies in real markets is far from conditions of perfect competition. If some people have more money than others, they can push up the price of a scarce good. This gives them preferential access to it and prevents others from being able to afford it, except at the cost of sacrificing the opportunity to acquire other goods. Similarly, producers limit access to goods specifically in order to be able to get a better price for them, or they undercut their rivals by reducing prices to force them out of business. By no means all producers have equal access to information about supply and demand. Ultimately, government may interfere with the market by deciding that a good should be available to all or that its production needs controlling. Once again this makes market freedom unrealisable in societies in which consumers have very unequal access to all the resources and information needed to make free market purchasing decisions.

Key questions

What social factors do you think may limit access to health care in:

- antenatal care;
- community services for old people;
- routine surgery;
- mental health services?

Health policies

The fundamental economic principles we have outlined frame the delivery of health care in most advanced industrial societies. Neither through free markets nor through rationing can all people be guaranteed equal treatment. For political reasons responses to such problems are often not addressed openly. The economic dilemmas represent structural constraints which cannot be ignored. Whether market or rationing mechanisms are adopted is essentially a policy decision. The key analytical questions are as follows.

1. Who decides on the allocation of health resources?

Should central government determine the full range of services to be provided by a national health system? They usually hold the most accurate national and international data about health trends and should be best placed to determine the epidemiological consequences of health allocation policies, taking a wider view of the needs of the whole society.

Should more localised authorities take decisions about resources given their detailed knowledge of the needs of the local population? National data are collected regionally. Providing information at a local level and through local representatives enables a direct response to the environmental and cultural determinants of health care. Such authorities might be health service managers who work daily with the relevant data.

Should allocation decisions be taken by individual clinicians? They are, after all, working with a more direct understanding of what is needed to meet their clients' requirements. In any case doctors and nurses already make rationing decisions. They ration the time they give to patients, the number of diagnostic procedures applied, the drugs they prescribe, the patients' length of stay in hospital and the care they allocate to patients according to combined personal and professional judgements about who deserves their attention.

Should the decision-makers be chosen by election or by appointment? If they are chosen by election, it is important to know what constituency they represent. If chosen by appointment, there would be questions about who should make such appointments and using what criteria. If we want to rely on impartial, specialist professional judgement, we may well prefer not to have clinicians elected by popular vote. There has to be a mechanism by which they are selected and appointed by their peers and superiors, who are best able to judge their professional expertise.

Health service managers should probably be similarly appointed, according to prior evidence of their ability to manage large organisations. Consequently, responsibility for monitoring professional accountability for action would lie solely with executive boards which supervise professional decisions and devise policy. Other members of such boards may be elected or appointed according to the experience they can bring to bear and to represent the outside interests of clients and the general population.

Some some balance between decisions taken at national, regional and client level must inevitably be reached. That balance entails a **tension between professional dominance and political patronage** in conferring decision-taking positions at both local and national levels. If clients became the ultimate decision-makers on service delivery, there would then have to be complete trust in the ability of a market to provide all that is required.

2. What principles will inform decisions on resource allocation?

Before rationing is determined **priorities have to be set.** Since not all problems can be addressed at once decisions have to be taken about which problems to deal with first. Such decisions may be based on pressing social needs such as the fear of an epidemic, illness or disease which threatens large numbers of the population. Conditions are often prioritised on the grounds that something can actually be done about them, that results can be measured and successful outcomes achieved, whereas other problems, perceived as insurmountable, may be neglected.

As with many economic decisions, some form of cost–benefit analysis will be used. The level of costs of certain actions will be weighed against their benefits. Such an approach will call into question why resources should be spent on someone whose **quality of life** has deteriorated so much that they can gain no pleasure from it. Alternatively, estimations of the opportunity cost or the marginal cost can be used to determine policy. **Opportunity cost** approaches can lead to decisions to treat young rather than old people on the basis that the latter have already benefited from and contributed to society all that they can, while the potential contribution of younger people – estimated in future years – may be much greater. **Marginal cost** approaches entail comparing the increase in unit costs of detecting and treating disease for each extra unit of population screened or treated. This may lead to decisions to limit screening or treatment to the highest-risk groups or not to screen at all on the grounds that it will make no estimable difference.

Decisions may be also based on estimations of **responsibility,** as discussed in Chapter 11. This would place a lower priority on a condition seen as self-inflicted or a consequence of actions for which the patient could be held responsible. Within a number of countries, notably the USA, it is increasingly likely that such a case may not be treated, or only be treated if consumers do not deprive others of the scarce service or if they pay for the service themselves.

Transferring costs

Another way of reducing health costs, at least on paper, is to redefine them as non-health and transfer them to non-health agencies. In Britain this has been adopted in community care reforms, which have seen a sizeable transfer of resources from health to social services. Simultaneously, the NHS has been placed under enormous political pressure to reduce waiting lists for hospital beds, causing an emphasis on discharging patients from acute hospital facilities.

There has not been a simple shift from health services to social services, as the nature of those social services, too, has been rapidly changing. The role of local social services departments as providers is changing to a focus on commissioning services. A private care sector has been largely created through a benefits-led expansion of private long-stay residential and nursing home care. Between the 1980s and 90s the number of local authority owned homes was halved. Over this same period the number of private sector homes increased threefold. The nursing care of older people initially shifted from geriatric wards in hospitals to nursing homes. Then the funds for nursing home care were transferred in the 1990s to social services. Boundary shifts caused by conflicting pressures on health and social services organisations have led to the redefinition of long-term health needs as '**social care**'. This justifies leaving them to be resourced through social services.

Health care system

The organisation of the British health care system currently mixes rationing with free market principles following NHS reforms of the 1980s and 90s. These were aimed at reducing the role of the state in managing both the economy and welfare provision in favour of an expansion of private, market competition. A strategy of privatisation and commodification was intended to promote the role of the market.

In order to construct a more price-competitive market some local health and social services have been designated as having a **purchaser** role, while professional health carer agencies have been designated as **provider** units which compete for purchasers' business. These developments have been accompanied by a central government framework of policy and legislation setting **health priority areas** for special attention. In effect an artificial market was established, government intervening artificially to establish 'demand' by setting priorities.

The emphasis on market principles in the early stages of NHS reform led to the appointment of managers with commercial experience but less understanding of public service. Senior executives and board members were appointed according to their political allegiances and their support of market principles. This tendency to run health care like a private business encouraged a system of patronage, greater secrecy in decision-making and information-gathering, and less public accountability.

The devolution of fundholding from central to local decision-makers also moved the responsibility for rationing care from a governmental body to a local health care professional. There is now a system of selective general practitioner (primary care physician) fundholding in Britain. This encourages decision-making on care to be based on what funds are made available to purchase services. Thus local providers have increasingly to adjust the services they provide according to what services have become financially viable rather than in response to patient needs.

Clinical effectiveness

The pressure for treatments to be cost-sensitive has increased the demand for evidence to be provided of their comparative levels of **clinical effectiveness**. Recent developments in **evidence-based practice** through monitoring the continued application of research findings to treatments offers a route to applying marginal costs principles in choosing treatments.

For example, evidence suggests that there may be extensive overprescribing of expensive drugs, that some routinely conducted gynaecological interventions have no proven benefit, that many radiographic investigations may be unnecessary, and that genetic and biomedical innovations may remove the need for expensive invasive medical treatments such as surgery.

Exercise

List the procedures which you have heard of or assisted with which you believe to cost more than is necessary. What criteria are you using to estimate 'necessary' and 'unnecessary' costs?

Use your list to suggest procedures or practices which you think would save money. Now think about how far these would involve prioritising some patients' needs rather than others or prioritising some types of need rather than others. How might these needs be met?

Consequences of policy developments

In moving longer-term care from hospitals and local authorities into the community considerable resources have been shifted to a complex of private care agencies and residential and nursing homes. The UK government also attempted to shift the funding of health services to private health insurance and a private commercial care sector through income tax cuts. However, such policies have incompletely addressed the needs of those groups most affected by the recessions, namely the poorer groups in society most likely to need health and welfare support. These groups are in no position to benefit from the kinds of change entailed in reconstructing health and welfare provision. The experiences of a wide number of social groups, including women, older people and professional carers, have consolidated a tide of public opinion in favour of continuing public provision of health and welfare services.

To counteract such opinions, Conservative governments have deployed ideologies which attempt to explain the health care problems of the disadvantaged in terms which would define them as having been morally responsible for those problems. Such ideologies include explaining higher levels of morbidity among poorer groups by highlighting lifestyle choices rather than, for example, housing problems. Using these kinds of explanation would also justify restricting their access to certain kinds of medical treatment. If families are seen as wholly responsible for health, individuals' rights to health care are less likely to be secured by their citizenship. Instead, access is far more likely to be subject to the inequalities of family wealth.

However, considerable controversy, indicating widespread disagreement with ideologies of individual rather than state responsibility, has been caused by the UK government charging the costs of the continuing health care of older people in nursing homes, once met by health authorities, to those people themselves. In many instances this has meant the disappearance of life savings and homes which may previously have been passed on in family inheritances. This is a major change in which middle-class groups have also been hit by care costs affecting their levels of support for government policies.

Setting up health care as more clearly based on contracts and consumerism has also brought the wider development of procedures for users to bring complaints against unsatisfactory services. The level of both formal complaints and litigation within the courts has risen sharply since the 1980s.

One consequence of basing services on individually negotiated contracts with a variety of care agencies has been the loss of integrated specialist services for specific groups such as children and the elderly. Deploying professional skills in more flexible general ways, combined with fewer resources, has increased disagreement between health and social services professionals about responsibility. Resolving the contradictions in state welfare remains a formidable obstacle (Offe 1984).

Public health

A number of professional health associations have suggested that public health would be well served by more co-ordination of services, and primary care staffing, especially in relation to specific social groups, would improve access for those currently disadvantaged. They have also suggested that there must be better record-keeping in relation to health inequalities.

The publication of the Black Report (Townsend and Davidson 1982) and the Health Inequalities Report (Whitehead 1987) achieved the aim of highlighting health inequalities in Britain and the role of structural factors in contributing to the pattern of health problems. Their recommendations were resisted as too expensive. However, Health Education Councils and medical associations, together with a variety of other allies such as church and voluntary groups, have collaborated to place multiple deprivation and health inequalities on the public agenda. This perspective underlining social influences on health has been further supported by activities following the World Health Organization Healthy Cities and Health For All initiatives (World Health Organization 1986).

A co-ordinated approach would call for more, rather than less, government policy-making in health and social services. It also means responding in a more co-ordinated way to the health implications of a variety of policies on work, housing, transport and leisure. There is increasing strain on the insurance-funded health facilities in the USA, with doubts about their effectiveness and ability to cope with increasing demands. Other countries have tackled health inequalities through a broader systematic approach. In Denmark inequalities in infant health have been reduced through intensive public health programmes linked to improved maternity benefits. In an attempt to influence international health outcomes by structural changes, food pricing policies in Norway have been used to stabilise world food supplies through decreasing imports, while encouraging dietary changes.

Conclusion

Public surveys in the UK have shown that, in 1977, one-third of those interviewed blamed the poor for their own problems. In contrast by 1986 more than half blamed circumstances beyond their control. Three-quarters thought that the rich–poor gap was 'too great' and supported increases in benefits through taxes. This indicates a renewal of interest in public health, an interest in strengthening health rather than reducing disease and widespread public support for retaining the British welfare state.

By the time you read this book a new Labour government will have been in power for some time in the UK. Many of the problematic policies discussed in this chapter drew on Conservative Party ideology and were implemented by a government which had held power for eighteen years. It will be interesting to see how the new government addresses the dilemmas of state welfare policies, but no state can afford to meet the full demand for health services which occurs in a modern society. **Priority-setting** is inevitable in health care. We have stressed the interconnectedness between all the social factors which influence health requirements. The difficulty in setting priorities is in deciding where public funds would be best allocated. Improvements in housing, work and education will all improve health. To seek to **apportion scarce resources to illness is to treat the symptom rather than the causes** of many health problems. Yet not to spend enough on symptoms is politically and morally unacceptable.

Key questions

This is the hardest question we have set – even governments struggle to answer it – but, given the principles outlined in this chapter:

How would you balance the allocation of both the scarce resources of the state and of the individual toward health care? Neither have unlimited amounts to spend, so how should the balance between spending on health – for the state and for households – be determined?

Further reading

Bywaters, P. and McLeod, E. (eds) (1996) *Working for Equality in Health*, London: Routledge.
    Written by practitioners, this book outlines strategies for combatting the health care effects of inequality in all its forms.

Green, D.G. (1996) *Community Without Politics: A Market Approach to Welfare Reform*, London: IEA Health and Welfare Unit.

Klein, R. and Day, P. (1996) *Managing Scarcity: Priority Setting and Rationing in the NHS*, Buckingham: Open University Press.
    In a conceptually difficult area, these books are both clear and thorough concerning the general principles involved.

Chapter 15 Modelling Health Care Sociologically

In previous chapters we have examined ways in which social processes create patterns of empowerment or disempowerment, inclusion or exclusion, visibility or invisibility, and can structure inequalities. We began with general sociological insights and built a more detailed analytical understanding of ways in which such patterns are reflected in experiences of health and illness, health work and health outcomes. We now put the pieces of the jigsaw together to construct a sociological map for the area within which humans experience health and illness.

Modelling health and illness

Health and illness are at either end of a **continuum**. At one end you would be 100 per cent healthy. At the other end you would be 100 per cent ill, that is, presumably, dead. This means that health and illness are not dichotomous concepts. People do not have absolute health or absolute illness but have some of both at any one time. Even individuals who are extremely healthy can be carrying illness-developing disease entities such as bacteria, viruses or cancer cells. Anyone may have organs that are not functioning optimally or an individual may simply 'not feel well'. Similarly, someone who is defined as ill may not be so ill that they cannot engage in some behaviour seen as healthy. People who have a cold may still do their daily exercise. People who are terminally ill do not necessarily lose their interest in sexual activity.

We have shown how sociology can uncover the variety of **social influences** that move people along this continuum towards health or illness. We have grouped such influences under headings such as class, gender and ethnicity to indicate that an individual's position on the health/illness continuum is influenced by occupation, status, power, income, wealth, language, cultural practices, values, norms and beliefs. We use these categories to consider whether particular social classes, occupations, genders or ethnic groupings are more or less likely to be exposed to specific health problems or more or less likely to be able to take effective steps to gain health resources or reduce health problems.

The problem in modelling movement along the health/illness continuum is to discover precisely how these influences affect the individual, whether singly or in combination. If they act in combination, we may also want to know more precisely how they interact with one another. Thus any model we construct would have to be based on rigorous investigation into the influence of these variables, both separately and together. We lack the space for such detail here, but we shall consider a few of the problems sociological researchers face in answering such a complex question.

Estimating the 'weight' of social influences

As we outlined in Chapter 1 there are a range of commonly recognised problems for sociological enquiry and explanations, including:

- how to measure human actions and meanings;
- predicting human behaviour;
- observing and experimenting with human groups;
- identifying and understanding people's reasons for their behaviour;
- the multiplicity of causes for social phenomena;
- the need to use 'probability' in causal statements.

To put our jigsaw together and find out what moves individuals along the health/illness continuum requires some estimation of the importance of such diverse influences. Official statistics offer useful data on health issues, but we have to remain alert to their limitations. Statistics are produced for the purposes of particular organisations and not necessarily for the plain seeking of facts. No continuous national survey of health and illness is available. Inferences about levels of health and illness have to be made on the basis of statistics produced for many other purposes.

Mortality statistics are not measures of illness: they are an outcome of what is considered by coroners to be an acceptable cause of death. Statistics on the uptake of health facilities are partial, dependent on those who have brought their condition to health service attention. Others who, for example, deal with their illness themselves or cannot afford the time for illness are excluded from the statistics. Sickness absence statistics neglect the unemployed, the part-time employed (the majority of working women), all those above and below employment age and absences too brief to be registered. The UK General Household Survey periodically asked a sample of the population directly about their health. Chronic illness was defined in terms of activity limitations compared with others of the same age. Long-term illness was defined relative to restrictions on the respondents' own usual activity. The flaw in this is evident, depending as it does on ideas of what counts as normal, everyday life.

All sociological research faces a problem of 'gate-keeping'. Agencies who control the access to data and respondents favour certain research approaches. Most social research depends upon gaining such access. Public health officials and medical practitioners often have to be persuaded of the validity of qualitative research techniques based on interactionist sociological perspectives. They may have had little experience of these techniques, given the dominance of laboratory-based or experimental methods in their own training. In addition, a disadvantage of welfare systems with fewer state regulations is that health care agencies frequently restrict or prevent the collection of data which allow unfavourable comparisons between providers. Cuts in public health monitoring make it more difficult to find appropriate categories of statistical data or even allow access to any politically sensitive data.

Estimating the success of policies depends upon the measurability of their outcomes. In health care certain outcome measures are easier to gather than others. Health status is notoriously difficult to measure (Hunt *et al.* 1985). More easily measured items, such as hospital treatment waiting lists, the number of particular surgical interventions, the numbers of patients admitted and discharged, and patient satisfaction ratings, are frequently regarded as key success indicators. Yet, as we have suggested, most of these are methodologically flawed as accurate indicators of service success.

Key questions

What measures of health status have you come across?

What agencies collect them?

Why do they collect them?

What aspects of how their collection affect their accuracy as measures of health:

- for a local population;
- for users of the agencies collecting these measures;
- for the general population?

Social epidemiology

Despite these reservations large-scale statistical data sets have become vital to an important branch of the sociological study of health and illness: that of social epidemiology. This is the study of the characteristics of groups of people in order to seek explanations of the incidences and prevalence of morbidity and mortality for those groups. Epidemiology uses quantitative indicators of these characteristics and draws conclusions which are dependent on assumed correlations between them. It grew out of the study of epidemics of infectious diseases (cholera, plague and influenza). More recently, it has been applied to cancer and heart disease.

Members of a population or comparative populations are counted according to certain physical, physiological or socio-demographic base data such as cholesterol levels, blood pressure, blood sugar counts, height, weight, ethnicity, gender, age, social class, marital status, housing arrangements, geographic area of residence and so on. The incidence and prevalence of any diseases or disorders are then counted for the same population(s). The counting must be repeated over a period of time and, preferably, comparatively with other populations in order to compare fluctuations in incidence and prevalence with changes in background characteristics of the population (Eyles and Woods 1983).

To take an example, various cancers have been assumed to be caused by smoking as a result of studies of populations of similar characteristics except that one group smokes and the other does not. The smoking group develops more cases of cancer. Each group has to be 'controlled' for as many identifiable factors as possible in order to exclude any other possible causes of the incidence. The first work showing conclusively the link between smoking and cancer was published in 1963 by one of the country's most eminent epidemiologists, Sir Richard Doll.

Epidemiological study points to the importance of statistical averages in the measurement of public health risk and leads to a focus on the distributions of morbidity and mortality within populations. As Jones and Moon (1987) demonstrate epidemiology provides a contrasting picture of health and illness to that adopted by clinical medicine. A doctor's need to classify and treat an illness, backed by the research evidence of clinical trials, leads to a health/illness dichotomy: if you are sick, you need assistance in the form of diagnosis, treatment and prognosis; if you are well, you do not need help. However, just as the individual does not experience health and illness dichotomously, so neither is the population composed of people who are either well or ill. The distribution of health and illness is continuous throughout the population. Thus, for example, there is no sudden change from those who have normal blood pressure to those whose blood pressure is abnormally high: blood pressure varies in degree between the extremes.

In terms of public health strategy this health/illness continuum is of significance. Extremes in the distribution are affected by the average. Thus the number of people with hypertension in a given population is predicted by the average blood pressure of the community. Similarly, the number of alcohol abusers in a population is predicted by the alcohol consumption of the average person in the population. As Bunton and Macdonald (1992) show a preferred health-promotion strategy would have everyone change a little rather than those at the extremes changing a lot; it would be easier to accomplish, less costly in terms of resources and likely to have longer-term effects. This challenges the usual methods for measuring the success of a health service. It may be less important for public health to attempt to reduce waiting lists or improve the delivery of health care; instead of targeting those who are already ill, it is better to prevent the rate of illness rising in the first place.

Epidemiology answers questions such as 'Why did this disease occur?' and 'Could it have been prevented?' These are just as important as asking 'What is the diagnosis?' and 'What should be the treatment?'

We have to exercise caution because the indicators employed are dependent on the ability accurately to quantify morbidity, mortality and health. The causes of disease cannot be proven by this means; they can only be assumed on the basis of adequate **correlation**. Correlation suggests an 'association' between several factors but not how particular outcomes might be caused by certain factors. Some of the difficulties of doing this in the UK can be estimated by looking at health-related statistical data published by the Office of National Statistics (formerly the Central Statistical Office). Look, for example, at the annual publication *Social Trends*.

Key questions

What would you routinely measure in order to link particular disease outcomes to the specific characteristics of populations or communities?

What difficulties would you anticipate in the collection of that data?

Epidemiology is macro-sociological in its focus upon populations rather than individuals. As with all macro-sociological data it omits the real experience of the meeting between health professionals and clients.

Professional/client encounters

The professional and client are each separately influenced by their role, status, cultural and community background, social class, family background, age, gender, education and qualifications. Their relationship, where they meet and overlap, is influenced by how each of these factors relates to the others. There are relative class, age, gender and status relationships which determine the power differentials between professional and client. Porter (1993), for example, looks at the effects of racism in such a setting.

How these influences combine to determine outcomes requires the addition of factors which condition the setting. These include the physical ecology of the room (surgery or clinic), institutional arrangements for the payment of fees, communication processes and the formal organisational arrangements for the meeting. Contextual influences include physical locations, social institutions and social groups. Particular contexts provide characteristically different kinds of social activity and language. It is by exploring these different **contexts for action** that we begin to make sense of what may first appear to us as inexplicable behaviour.

Exercise

Using all the analytic tools recommended so far, conduct a sociological analysis of any professional/client encounter you have experienced. Think about power differentials, relative roles and role conflicts, and background forms of structured inequality. On the basis of your analysis consider the range of possible outcomes to the encounter. Are some outcomes more likely than others?

We have offered you some of the tools available within sociology for conducting such analyses. To encourage direct applications to your own experiences we have presented some areas of theory and research as less 'problematic' than they are. Life and society are always changing. Sociologists do not always necessarily agree upon ways of understanding the world. Research is ongoing and it is up to you, as sociologically aware health care professionals, to pursue the further reading and references suggested. In this way you will extend the routes to reflect on action that we have presented.

Conclusion: Understanding experiences

By now you have acquired an overview of how we come to understand the individuated experience of health and illness. Everyone constructs **lay models** to interpret the experience of health and of illness. They are formed from **concepts** (feelings, thoughts, attitudes and perceptions) and **behaviour** (actions, habits and practices) which emerge out of the social processes directly conditioning experiences of health and illness. Such processes include the accidents of history, geography, biology and biography which intersect with individual lives; these are the unique events that happen to us and they colour our personal perspectives. However, such social processes are contained within the material, cultural and political constraints (or potential liberations) of social structures. This structural framework conditions our unique experiences and produces the patterned outcomes we see in health policies and health care treatment.

Our investigative, analytic theme is designed to expand the **expert model** and encourage a holist perspective. The sociologically informed expert model must transcend any immediate individuated experience, highlight significant aspects of that experience and demonstrate its origins and consequences. It must be interdisciplinary, making connections between structural and processual conditions. People are social, psychological and biological creatures surviving in a physical and biochemical universe. Sociology offers only a part of the picture that aids our understanding of how that survival is made possible.

Further reading

The following books look in detail at the difficulties of measuring and modelling health and illness, and make comparison with other countries:

Gray, A. and Payne, P. (1993) *World Health and Disease*, Health and Disease Series, Book 3, Buckingham: Open University Press.

Kaplan, R.M., Sallis, J.F. and Patterson, T.L. (1993) *Health and Human Behavior*, New York: McGraw-Hill.

Lafaille, R. and Fulder, S. (eds) (1993) *Towards a New Science of Health*, London: Routledge.

McConway, K. (ed.) (1994) *Studying Health and Disease*, Buckingham: Open University Press.

References

Abbott, P. and Wallace, C. (1990) *An Introduction to Sociology: Feminist Perspectives*, London: Routledge.

Adler, N.E., Kegeles, S.M. and Genevro, J.L. (1992) 'Risk taking and health' Chapter 8, pp. 231–55 in Yates, J.F. (ed.) *Risk-Taking Behaviour*, Chichester: John Wiley & Sons.

Arber, S. and Ginn, J. (1992) 'Research note – class and caring: a forgotten dimension', *Sociology*, **26**: 619–34.

Baron-Cohen, S. (1995) *Mindblindness*, London: MIT Press/Bradford Books.

Bateson, M.C. (1989) *Composing a Life*, New York: Plume.

Becker, G. and Nachtigall, R.D. (1992) 'Eager for medicalisation: the social production of infertility as a disease', *Sociology of Health and Illness*, **14**: 456–71.

Becker, H.S. (1961) *Boys in White: Student Culture in Medical School*, Chicago: University of Chicago Press.

Becker, H.S. (1963) *Outsiders*, New York: Free Press.

Belbin, M. (1981) *Management Teams: Why They Succeed or Fail*, London: Heinemann.

Benner, P. (1984) 'Excellence and power in clinical nursing practice', Chapter 14, pp. 207–20 in Benner, P. *From Novice to Expert: Excellence and Power in Clinical Nursing Practice*, California: Addison-Wesley.

Benzeval, M., Judge, K. and Smaje, C. (1995) 'Beyond class, race and ethnicity – deprivation and health in Britain', *Health Services Research*, **30**: 163–77.

Bernstein, B. (1975) *Class, Codes and Control* (vol. 1), London: Routledge & Kegan Paul.

Blane, D., Brunner, E. and Wilkinson, R. (1996) *Health and Social Organization*, London: Routledge.

Blaxter, M. (1996) 'The significance of socioeconomic factors in health for medical care and the National Health Service', Chapter 3, pp. 32–41 in Blane, D., Brunner, E. and Wilkinson, R., *Health and Social Organization*, London: Routledge.

Booth, C. (1889) *Life and Labour of the People in London*, London: Williams & Norgate.

References

Bott, E. (1971) *Family and Social Network* (2nd edn), London: Tavistock.
Braithwaite, R. and Lythcott, N. (1989) 'Community empowerment as a strategy for health promotion for black and other minorities', *Journal of the American Medical Association*, **261**: 282–3.
Braverman, H. (1974) *Labour and Monopoly Capital: The Degradation of Work in the Twentieth Century*, New York: Monthly Review Press.
Brown, C. and Jasper, K. (eds) (1993) *Consuming Passions: Feminist Approaches to Eating Disorders and Weight Preoccupations*, Toronto: Second Story Press.
Bunton, R. and Macdonald, G. (eds) (1992) *Health Promotion: Disciplines and Diversity*, London: Routledge.
Bywaters, P. and McLeod, E. (1996) *Working for Equality in Health*, London: Routledge.
Carpenter, M. (1996) 'Beyond "us and them": trade unions and equality in community care for users and workers', Chapter 9, pp. 124–39 in Bywaters, P. and McLeod, E., *Working for Equality in Health*, London: Routledge.
Checkland, P. (1981) *Systems Thinking and Systems Practice*, Chichester: John Wiley & Sons.
Chrisman, N.J. (1977) 'The health-seeking process: an approach to the natural history of illness', *Culture, Medicine and Psychiatry*, **1**: 351–77.
Cohen, S. (1971) *Images of Deviance*, Harmondsworth: Penguin.
Cooper, C. (1996) 'Hot under the collar', *Times Higher Education Supplement*, June 21, p. 15.
Cooper, D. (1972) *The Death of the Family*, Harmondsworth: Penguin.
Corrigan, P. (1979) *Schooling the Smash Street Kids*, London: Macmillan.
Cousins, C. (1987) *Controlling Social Welfare: A Sociology of State Welfare Work and Organisation*, Brighton: Harvester Wheatsheaf.
Culley, L. (1996) 'A critique of multiculturalism in health-care – the challenge for nurse education', *Journal of Advanced Nursing*, **23**: 564–70.
Dahl, R.A. (1984) *Modern Political Analysis* (4th edn), New Jersey: Prentice-Hall .
Davey, B., Gray, A. and Seale, C. (eds) (1995) *Health and Disease: A Reader* (2nd edn), Buckingham: Open University Press.
Davies, C. (1995) *Gender and the Professional Predicament in Nursing*, Buckingham: Open University Press.
Davis, K. and Moore, W.E. (1967) 'Some principles of stratification' in Bendix, R. and Lipset, S.M. (eds), *Class, Status and Power* (2nd edn) London: Routledge & Kegan Paul.
Deem, R. (1986) *All Work and No Play: The Sociology of Women and Leisure*, Milton Keynes: Open University Press.
Douglas, M. (1973) *Natural Symbols (Explorations in Cosmology)* (2nd edn), London: Barrie and Jenkins.
Douglas, M. (1992) *Risk and Blame (Essays in Cultural Theory)*, London: Routledge.

Doyal, L. (1995) *What Makes Women Sick: Gender and the Political Economy of Health*, London: Macmillan.

Durkheim, E. (1895/1947) *The Division of Labour in Society*, New York: Free Press.

Eyles, J. and Woods, K.J. (1983) *The Social Geography of Medicine and Health*, London: Croom Helm.

Fagot, B.I. (1984) *Early sex role development: gender identity and adoption of sex-typed behaviors* (audio sound cassette), CSWS Speaker Series; Lecture presented 17 January 1984 at the University of Oregon for the Center for the Study of Women in Society.

Field, F. (1989) *Losing Out*, Oxford: Blackwell.

Finch, J. (1989) *Family Obligations and Social Change*, Cambridge: Polity Press.

Finerman, R. and Bennett, L.A. (1995) 'Guilt, blame and shame: responsibility in health and sickness', *Social Science and Medicine*, **40**: 1–3.

Fischer, C.S. (1976) 'Alienation: trying to bridge the chasm', *British Journal of Sociology*, **27**: 35–47.

Foucault, M. (1973) *The Birth of the Clinic: An Archaeology of Medical Perception*, trans. A.M. Sheridan Smith, London: Tavistock.

Friedson, E. (1994) *Professionalism Reborn: Theory, Prophecy and Policy*, Cambridge: Polity Press.

Gabe, J. (ed.) (1995) *Medicine, Health and Risk*, Oxford: Blackwell.

Gabe, J., Kelleher, D. and Williams, G. (eds) (1994) *Challenging Medicine*, London: Routledge.

Giddens, A. (1997) *Sociology* (3rd edn), Cambridge: Polity Press.

Goffman, E. (1959) *The Presentation of Self in Everyday Life*, London: Penguin.

Goffman, E. (1968a, reprinted 1990) *Stigma: Notes on the Management of Spoiled Identity*, Harmondsworth: Penguin.

Goffman, E. (1968b) *Asylums*, Harmondsworth: Penguin.

Goffman, E. (1979) *Gender Advertisements*, London: Macmillan.

Goldthorpe, J. (1983) 'Women and class analysis: in defence of the conventional view', *Sociology*, **17**: 465–87.

Graham, H. (1984) *Women, Health and the Family*, Brighton: Harvester Wheatsheaf.

Graham, H. (1993) *Hardship and Health in Women's Lives*, Brighton: Harvester Wheatsheaf.

Halmos, P. (1970) *The Personal Service Society*, London: Constable.

Handy, C.B. (1989) *The Age of Unreason*, London: Business Books.

Haralambos, M. and Holborn, M. (1991) *Sociology: Themes and Perspectives* (3rd edn), London: Collins Educational.

Hayes, R.H., Wheelwright, S.C. and Clark, K.B. (1988) *Dynamic Manufacturing: Creating the Learning Organization*, New York: Free Press.

Hunt, S.M., McEwen, J., and McKenna, S.P. (1985) 'Measuring health status: a new tool for clinicians and epidemiologists', *Journal of the Royal College of General Practitioners*, **35**: 185–8.

Iphofen, R. (1990) 'Coping with a "perforated life": a case study in managing the stigma of petit mal epilepsy', *Sociology*, **24**: 447–63.

James, N. (1989) 'Care = organisation + physical labour + emotional labour', *Sociology of Health and Illness*, **14**: 488–509.

Jones, K. and Moon, G. (1987) *Health, Disease and Society: A Critical Medical Geography*, London: Routledge & Kegan Paul.

Kaplan, R.M., Sallis, J.F. and Patterson, T.L. (1993) *Health and Human Behavior*, New York: McGraw-Hill.

Kuhn, A. (1985) *The Power of the Image – Essays on Representation and Sexuality*, London: Routledge & Kegan Paul.

Labov, W. (1969) 'The logic of nonstandard English', pp. 283–307 in Giglioli, P.P. (ed.) (1972) *Language and Social Context*, Harmondsworth: Penguin.

Laing, R.D. (1967) *The Politics of Experience and the Bird of Paradise*, Harmondsworth: Penguin.

Laing, R.D. (1969) *The Divided Self*, New York: Pantheon.

Laing, R.D. (1971) *Self and Others* (2nd edn), Harmondsworth: Penguin.

Laing, R.D. and Esterson, A. (1970) *Sanity, Madness and the Family*, Harmondsworth: Penguin.

Laslett, P. (1977) 'Characteristics of the Western family considered over time', *Journal of Family History*, **2**: 89–114.

Lawler, J. (1991) *Behind the Screens: Nursing, Somology and the Problem of the Body*, London: Churchill Livingstone.

Leach, Sir Edmund (1967) BBC Reith Lectures.

Lemert, E. (1972) *Human Deviance, Social Problems and Social Control*, Englewood Cliffs, NJ: Prentice-Hall.

Lewis, O. (1961) *The Children of Sanchez*, London: Secker & Warburg.

Lister, I. (ed.) (1974) *Deschooling: A Reader*, London: Cambridge University Press.

Littlewood, R. and Lipsedge, M. (1989) *Aliens and Alienists: Ethnic Minorities and Psychiatry*, London: Routledge (Unwin Hyman).

Lukes, S. (1974) *Power: A Radical View*, London: Macmillan.

Mann, M. (1992) *The Making of an English 'Underclass'?* Milton Keynes: Open University.

Marmot, M. and Feeney, A. (1996) 'Work and health: implications for individuals and society', Chapter 13, pp. 235–54 in Blane, D., Brunner, E. and Wilkinson, R. *Health and Social Organization*, London: Routledge.

Marx, K. (1864/1970) *Capital* (vol. 1), London: Lawrence & Wishart.

Mayo, E. (1949) *The Social Problems of an Industrial Civilization*, London: Routledge & Kegan Paul.

Melia, K. (1987) *Learning and Working: The Occupational Socialisation of Nurses*, London: Tavistock.

Morgan, M. (1996) 'Perceptions and use of anti-hypertensive drugs among cultural groups', in Williams, S. J. and Calnan, M. (eds) *Modern Medicine*, London: UCL Press.

Sociology in Practice for Health Care Professionals

5Sociology *in Practice for Health Care Professionals*

Sociology in Practice for Health Care Professionals

Sociology in Practice for Health Care Professionals

Morris, D. (1989) 'Language and social networks in Ynys Mon', *Contemporary Wales*, 3: 99–117.

Morris, L. (1985) 'Renegotiation of the domestic division of labour in the context of male redundancy', pp. 400–16 in Roberts, B., Finegan, R. and Gallie, D. (eds) *New Approaches to Economic Life*, Manchester: Manchester University Press.

Murray, C. (1984) *Losing Ground: American Social Policy 1950–1980*, New York: Basic Books.

Murray, C. (1990) *The Emerging British Underclass*, London: Institute of Economic Affairs.

Nagler, M. (1993) 'The disabled: the acquisition of power', in Nagler, M. (ed.) *Perspective on Disability: Tests and Readings on Disability*, Palo Alto: Health Markets Research.

Neighbors, H.W., Braithwaite, R.L. and Thompson, E. (1995) 'Health promotion and African-Americans – from personal empowerment to community action', *American Journal of Health Promotion*, 9: 281–7.

Nightingale, F. (1860) *Suggestions for Thought to the Searchers after Truth Among the Artisans of England*, London: Eyre & Spottiswoode.

Oakley, A. (1974) *The Sociology of Housework*, Oxford: Martin Robertson.

Oakley, A. (1979) *Becoming a Mother*, Oxford: Martin Robertson.

Oakley, A. (1984) *The Captured Womb*, Harmondsworth: Penguin.

O'Brien, L.O. and Harris, F. (1991) *Retailing, Shopping, Society and Space*, London: Fulton Publishers.

Offe, C. (1984) *Contradictions of the Welfare State*, London: Hutchinson.

Open Systems Group (eds) (1981) *Systems Behaviour* (3rd edn), Milton Keynes: Open University.

Orbach, S. (1978) *Fat is a Feminist Issue*, New York: Paddington Press.

Packard, V. (1957) *The Hidden Persuaders*, London: Penguin.

Parsons, T. (1951) *The Social System*, New York: Free Press.

Payer, L. (1990) *Medicine and Culture: Notions of Health and Sickness*, London: Gollancz.

Peterson, C. (1995) 'Explanatory style and health', Chapter 14, pp. 233–46 in Buchanan, G.M. and Seligman, M.E.P. (eds) *Explanatory Style*, Hove: Lawrence Erlbaum Associates.

Poland, F. (1990) 'Breaking the rules: assessing the assessment of a girls' project', pp. 159–71 in Stanley, E. (ed.) *Feminist Praxis*, London: Routledge.

Poland, F. (1992) 'Trading relationships: home selling and petty enterprise in women's lives', pp. 175–89 in Arber, S. and Gilbert, N. (eds) *Women and Working Lives*, London: Macmillan.

Poland, F., Curran, M. and Owens, R.G. (1996) *Women and Senior Management: A Research Study of Career Barriers and Progression in the Library and Information Sector*, London: Library Association.

Porter, S. (1993) 'Critical realist ethnography: the case of racism and professionalism in a medical setting', *Sociology*, 27: 591–609.

References

Radley, A. (1994) *Making Sense of Illness: The Social Psychology of Health and Disease*, London: Sage.

Riska, E. and Wegar, K. (eds) (1993) *Gender, Work and Medicine*, London: Sage.

Rogers, W. Stainton (1991) *Explaining Health and Illness: An Exploration of Diversity*, Hemel Hempstead: Harvester Wheatsheaf.

Rose, H. and Rose, S. (1979) 'The IQ myth' Chapter 5, pp. 79–94 in Rubinstein, D., *Education and Equality*, Harmondsworth: Penguin.

Rose, P. and Platzer, H. (1993) 'Confronting prejudice... the nursing care of lesbians and gay men', *Nursing Times*, **89**: 52–4.

Rowntree, B.S. (1899) *Poverty: A Study of Town Life*, London: Macmillan.

Rubin, J.Z., Provenzano, F.J., and Luria, Z. (1974) 'The eye of the beholder: parents' views on the sex of newborns', *American Journal of Orthopsychiatry*, **44**: 512–19.

Rubinstein, D. (1979) *Education and Equality*, Harmondsworth: Penguin.

Runciman, W.G. (1972) *Relative Deprivation and Social Justice*, Harmondsworth: Penguin.

Scheff, T.J. (1966) *Being Mentally Ill: A Sociological Theory*, Chicago: Aldine.

Seeman, M. (1969) 'On the meaning of alienation', p. 150 in Coser, L.A. and Rosenberg, B. (eds) *Sociological Theory: A Book of Readings* (3rd edn), New York: Macmillan.

Seeman, M. and Lewis, S. (1995) 'Powerlessness, health and mortality: a longitudinal study of older men and mature women', *Social Science and Medicine*, **41**: 517–25.

Sharm, D. (1996) 'Attribution of blame for a child's disability', *Professional Nurse*, **11**: 790–2.

Smith, A. (1986) *The Ethnic Origins of Nations*, Oxford: Blackwell.

Smith, A. (1991) *National Identity*, Harmondsworth: Penguin.

Smith, C. and Lloyd, B.B. (1978) 'Maternal behaviour and perceived sex of infant', *Child Development*, **49**: 1263–5.

Smith, P. (1992) *The Emotional Labour of Nursing*, London: Macmillan.

Sontag, S. (1982) 'The pornographic imagination', in *A Susan Sontag Reader*, Harmondsworth: Penguin.

Stockwell, F. (1973) *The Unpopular Patient*, London: RCN.

Sutherland, E.H. (1949) *Principles of Criminology*, Chicago: J.B. Lippincott.

Suttles, G. (1972) *The Social Construction of Communities*, Chicago: University of Chicago Press.

Taylor, F.W. (1911/1947) *The Principles of Scientific Management*, New York: Harper & Row.

Telles, J.L. and Pollack, M.H. (1981) 'Feeling sick: the experience and legitimation of illness', *Social Science and Medicine*, **15A**: 243–51.

Thornton, P. and Lunt, N. (1995) *Employment for Disabled People: Social Obligation or Individual Responsibility?*, York: Social Policy Research Unit.

Townsend, P. (ed.) (1970) *The Concept of Poverty*, London: Heinemann.

Townsend, P. and Davidson, N. (1982) *Inequalities in Health: The Black Report*, Harmondsworth: Penguin.
United Nations (1996) *The Human Development Report*, Oxford University Press.
Walby, S. and Greenwell, J., with Mackay, L. and Soothill, K. (1994) *Medicine and Nursing: Professions in a Changing Health Service*, London: Sage.
Warner, M. (1987) *Monuments and Maidens: The Allegory of the Female Form*, London: Picador.
Weber, M. (1925) *Economy and Society: An Outline of Interpretive Sociology*, Roth, G. and Wittich, C. (eds) (1968), New York: Bedminster Press, a translation of *Wirtschaft und Gesellschaft. Grudriss der verstehenden Soziologie*, (1925) J.C.B. Mohr (P. Siebeck), Tubingen.
Weeks, J. (1981) *Sex, Politics and Society: The Regulation of Society Since 1800*, London: Longman.
Weiner, B. (1993) 'On sin versus sickness: a theory of perceived responsibility and social motivation', *American Psychologist*, **48**: 957–65.
Wenger, G.C. (1994) *Support Networks of Older People: A Guide for Practitioners*, Bangor: University of Wales, Centre for Social Policy Research and Development.
Whitehead, M. (1987) *The Health Divide: Inequalities in Health in the 1980s*, London: Health Education Council.
Whitehead, M. and Dahlgren, G. (1991) 'What can be done about inequalities in health?', *Lancet*, **338**: 1059–63.
Wilkins, L.T. (1965) *Social Deviance: Social Policy, Action, and Research*, London: Tavistock.
Williams, D.R. and Collins, C. (1995) 'US socio-economic and racial differences in health – patterns and explanations', *Annual Review of Sociology*, **21**: 349–86.
Wilson, W.J. (1978) *The Declining Significance of Race: Blacks and Changing American Institutions*, Chicago: University of Chicago Press.
Wolf, Naomi (1991) *The Beauty Myth*, Toronto: Vintage Books.
Woodward, J. (1965) *Industrial Organization: Theory and Practice*, London: Oxford University Press.
World Health Organization (1986) *Targets for Health for All*, Copenhagen: World Health Organization.
Young, M. and Willmott, P. (1961) *Family and Kinship in East London*, Harmondsworth: Penguin.
Young, M. and Willmott, P. (1975) *The Symmetrical Family*, Harmondsworth: Penguin.
Zola, I.K. (1972) 'Medicine as an institution of social control', *Sociological Review*, **20**: 487–504.
Zola, I. K. (1973) 'Pathways to the doctor – from person to patient', *Social Science and Medicine*, **7**: 677–89.

Index

M
macro-sociology, 13, 251
marginalisation, 168
marriage, 54
Marx, Karl, 10, 89, 130–1
Mead, George Herbert, 10
medicalisation, 151–3, 155–61, 176–8,
    185, 205
micro-sociology, 13
models of health and illness, 180–2,
    246–9, 253
moral panic, 208
multiculturalism, 172–3

N
normative structure, 43

O
occupational change, 105–6
oligarchy, 99
organic analogy, 9
organisations, 99–104
    virtual, 105

P
Parsons, Talcott, 9
peer groups, 34
phenomenology, 11
play, 36
political resources, 20–3
portfolio work, 105
postmodernism, 12
poverty, 117–28
    subculture, 125
power, 18–30, 136, 200–1
    devolved, 28
    limits, 29
    patient, 27, 50–2
priority-setting, 239–41, 244–5
professional/client relationship,
    49–50, 251–2
professionalisation, 97–100, 135
purchaser/provider, 236, 241

Q
quality of life, 239

R
race, 164
racism, 166
rationing, 235–7
reductionism, 5
relative deprivation, 122, 220
reproductive technology, 157–60
research problems, 247–9
responsibility, 188–90, 239–40
restricted codes, 77
risk, 140–1, 190
rites of passage, 34, 170–2

role, 37, 39–50
    complementarity, 50, 203
    conflict, 44
    distance, 44

S
Sacks, Harvey, 11
sanctions, 203–4
Schutz, Alfred, 11
scientific explanation, 1, 183–4
scientific management, 91
self-concept, 38–9
sexism, 145
sexuality, 160–1
sick role, 45–9
significant others, 40
social care, 240
social class, 130–42
social control agencies, 196, 210–12
social differentiation, 34
social distance, 201
social inequality, 109–28
    measurement, 111–15
social institutions, 9
socialisation, 32–6
    agencies, 33
    primary, 33
    secondary, 33, 68
social networks, 166–7, 169–70
social pathology, 195
social problems, 6
social status, 112–14
social stratification, 110
Spencer, Herbert, 9
stigma, 205–7, 217
structuralist perspective, 10
structuration theory, 12, 137
synergy, 101
systems theory, 9

T
team work, 102–3
theoretical perspectives, 7
total institution, 211

U
underclass, 124, 179
unemployment, 217–21

V
vocation, 89

W
wealth, 116–17, 135
Weber, Max, 89–90, 99, 131–2
welfare policy, 234–45
work, 87–107
    housework, 214–17
    women, 148–50